Understanding Ethics for Nursing Students

Sara Miller McCune founded SAGE Publishing in 1965 to support the dissemination of usable knowledge and educate a global community. SAGE publishes more than 1000 journals and over 800 new books each year, spanning a wide range of subject areas. Our growing selection of library products includes archives, data, case studies and video. SAGE remains majority owned by our founder and after her lifetime will become owned by a charitable trust that secures the company's continued independence.

Los Angeles | London | New Delhi | Singapore | Washington DC | Melbourne

2nd Edition

Understanding Ethics for Nursing Students

Peter Ellis

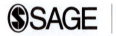

Learning Matters
An imprint of SAGE Publications Ltd
1 Oliver's Yard
55 City Road
London EC1Y 1SP

SAGE Publications Inc.
2455 Teller Road
Thousand Oaks, California 91320

SAGE Publications India Pvt Ltd
B 1/I 1 Mohan Cooperative Industrial Area
Mathura Road
New Delhi 110 044

SAGE Publications Asia-Pacific Pte Ltd
3 Church Street
#10-04 Samsung Hub
Singapore 049483

© Peter Ellis 2017
Chapter 2 © Lioba Howatson-Jones and Peter Ellis 2017
Chapter 7 © Peter Ellis and Hilary Engward 2017
Chapter 8 © Hilary Engward 2017

First edition published 2015
Second edition published 2017

Editor: Alex Clabburn
Development editor: Richenda Milton-Daws
Production controller: Chris Marke
Project management: Swales and Willis Ltd, Exeter, Devon
Marketing manager: Tamara Navaratnam
Cover design: Wendy Scott
Typeset by: C&M Digitals (P) Ltd, Chennai, India
Printed and bound by CPI Group (UK) Ltd, Croydon, CR0 4YY

Library of Congress Control Number: 2017936978

British Library Cataloguing in Publication data

A catalogue record for this book is available from the British Library

ISBN 978-1-4739-9788-2
ISBN 978-1-4739-9789-9 (pbk)

At SAGE we take sustainability seriously. Most of our products are printed in the UK using FSC papers and boards. When we print overseas we ensure sustainable papers are used as measured by the PREPS grading system. We undertake an annual audit to monitor our sustainability.

Contents

Transforming Nursing Practice is a series tailor-made for pre-registration student nurses. Each book in the series is:

○ Affordable
○ Mapped to the NMC Standards and Essential Skills Clusters
○ Full of active learning features
○ Focused on applying theory to practice

Each book addresses a core topic and has been carefully developed to be simple to use, quick to read and written in clear language.

"

An invaluable series of books that explicitly relates to the NMC standards. Each book covers a different topic that students need to explore in order to develop into a qualified nurse... I would recommend this series to all pre-registration nursing students whatever their field or year of study

Linda Robson
Senior Lecturer, Edge Hill University

The set of books is an excellent resource for students. The series is small, easily portable and valuable. I use the whole set on a regular basis.

Fiona Davies
Senior Nurse Lecturer, University of Derby

I recommend the SAGE/Learning Matters series to all my students as they are relevant and concise. Please keep up the good work.

Thomas Beary
Senior Lecturer in Mental Health Nursing, University of Hertfordshire

"

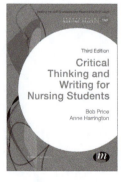

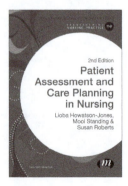

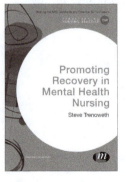

CORE KNOWLEDGE TITLES:

Becoming a Registered Nurse: Making the Transition to Practice
Communication and Interpersonal Skills in Nursing (3rd Ed)
Contexts of Contemporary Nursing (2nd Ed)
Getting into Nursing (2nd Ed)
Health Promotion and Public Health for Nursing Students (3rd Ed)
Introduction to Medicines Management in Nursing
Law and Professional Issues in Nursing (4th Ed)
Leadership, Management and Team Working in Nursing (2nd Ed)
Learning Skills for Nursing Students
Medicines Management in Children's Nursing
Microbiology and Infection Prevention and Control for Nursing Students
Nursing and Collaborative Practice (2nd Ed)
Nursing and Mental Health Care
Nursing in Partnership with Patients and Carers
Palliative and End of Life Care in Nursing
Passing Calculations Tests for Nursing Students (3rd Ed)
Pathophysiology and Pharmacology for Nursing Students
Patient Assessment and Care Planning in Nursing (2nd Ed)
Patient Safety and Managing Risk in Nursing
Psychology and Sociology in Nursing (2nd Ed)
Successful Practice Learning for Nursing Students (2nd Ed)
Understanding Ethics for Nursing Students (2nd Ed)
Understanding Psychology for Nursing Students
Using Health Policy in Nursing Practice
What is Nursing? Exploring Theory and Practice (3rd Ed)

PERSONAL AND PROFESSIONAL LEARNING SKILLS TITLES:

Clinical Judgement and Decision Making for Nursing Students (3rd Ed)
Critical Thinking and Writing for Nursing Students (3rd Ed)
Evidence-based Practice in Nursing (3rd Ed)
Information Skills for Nursing Students
Reflective Practice in Nursing (3rd Ed)
Succeeding in Essays, Exams and OSCEs for Nursing Students
Succeeding in Literature Reviews and Research Project Plans for Nursing Students (3rd Ed)

Successful Professional Portfolios for Nursing Students (2nd Ed)
Understanding Research for Nursing Students (3rd Ed)

MENTAL HEALTH NURSING TITLES:

Assessment and Decision Making in Mental Health Nursing
Critical Thinking and Reflection for Mental Health Nursing Students
Engagement and Therapeutic Communication in Mental Health Nursing
Medicines Management in Mental Health Nursing (2nd Ed)
Mental Health Law in Nursing
Physical Healthcare and Promotion in Mental Health Nursing
Promoting Recovery in Mental Health Nursing
Psychosocial Interventions in Mental Health Nursing

ADULT NURSING TITLES:

Acute and Critical Care in Adult Nursing (2nd Ed)
Caring for Older People in Nursing
Dementia Care in Nursing
Medicines Management in Adult Nursing
Nursing Adults with Long Term Conditions (2nd Ed)
Safeguarding Adults in Nursing Practice (2nd Ed)

You can find more information on each of these titles and our other learning resources at **www.sagepub.co.uk**. Many of these titles are also available in various e-book formats, please visit our website for more information.

About the authors

Peter Ellis is Head of Clinical Services at St Michael's Hospice, Hastings and Rother; prior to this he was Director of Nursing at Hospice in the Weald, Pembury. Peter is an Honorary Senior Research Fellow of Canterbury Christ Church University where he was a Senior Lecturer. Peter has degrees in Nursing, Ethics and Medical Epidemiology and has been writing for nurses for over 25 years, including three other books in the Transforming Nursing Practice series.

Hilary Engward is Senior Lecturer at Anglia Ruskin University. She teaches on post-registration Masters and PhD and Professional Doctoral courses. Hilary's background is in adult nursing. She has taught in universities since 2003, and has particular academic and research interests in healthcare ethics and medical and healthcare education.

Lioba Howatson-Jones was Senior Lecturer in Nursing and Applied Clinical Studies at Canterbury Christ Church University, until her recent retirement. Her clinical background has mainly been in acute nursing and practice development, and she has researched widely into nurses' learning. Lioba is the author of the book on Reflective Practice in this series and has contributed to other volumes.

Acknowledgements

To my girls, Jane, Emiliee and Hannah who are a constant inspiration. Also to all hospice staff and volunteers worldwide who selflessly give of themselves daily.

Introduction

Peter Ellis

In this book we attempt to introduce you to some of the ideas, concepts and realities of life as an ethical nurse. That is to say we take a very practical view of ethics rather than trying to present ethical thinking as something separate from the working lives of nurses and nursing students. This is very deliberate since we regard ethical thought and the exercise of ethics within practice to be as important as other nursing staples such as infection control.

We know from experience some students are challenged by the notion of ethics and what this means for them, their thinking as well as what is required of them in the work place by way of action. In this book we demonstrate to you not only why ethics is important, but also how ethics applies to your thinking and activity in the university, the practice setting and in day-to-day life; that is we consider ethicality in thought and action should play as an important part in our lives away from work as it does at work.

By default this book is very westernised in its approach to ethics: this is a result of the fact the authors have trained, worked and taught within a westernised model of healthcare and healthcare ethics. This should not be seen as us not appreciating that there are a number of world views of ethics; rather it reflects our experience and expertise, as well as the settings within which the majority of our readers will work.

Chapter 1 establishes the nature and purpose of ethics especially in how they apply to nursing and nursing students. We consider the nature of the establishment of identity as a nurse and the impact others have on the student nurse as you seek to develop an identity as a professional. We also examine the nature of values in nursing and what influence these have on the ways in which we develop our nursing identities and ways of working.

In the second chapter, initially written by Lioba and edited in this edition by Peter, we deviate from the norm for ethics textbooks in that we attempt to establish a mechanism for ethical thinking and decision making which establishes the importance of reflection in and on action. The important message within this chapter is that we need to allow ethical principles and concepts to drive our ethical decision making, rather than allowing our knee-jerk response to an ethical situation to drive us to look for ethical arguments to a decision we have made instinctively. The importance of embedding this inductive approach to ethical decision making is seen to parallel the better ways of employing evidence in our nursing practice. In some respects the new approach to revalidation for nurses underpins the importance of reflection on and in action. This is especially true in how it relates to practice issues which require us to reflect on the content of *The Code* both singularly and with others.

The third chapter explores some of the ideas of what ethics might be as well as exploding some of the myths. You are encouraged to explore your own understandings of the influences on your view of ethics and how these influences colour the ways in which you see the world and approach ethical decision making. This chapter therefore leads you, the reader, into a voyage of self-discovery, allowing you to examine what influences the nurse you choose to become.

Chapter 4 introduces some of the key approaches to ethics which influence western healthcare provision. These approaches are in turn influenced by the nature of intent, which is explored in some detail at the start of the chapter. Following on from this we introduce and explore some of the key elements of consequentialist, non-consequentialist and virtue ethics.

The discussion of rights, where they come from and how they might apply, is the subject matter of Chapter 5. Rights are pervasive in modern society, although many of us know very little about where they come from, what they require others to do, what privileges they confer on the holder and what happens when there appears to be a conflict of rights. This chapter seeks to explore some of these issues as well as examining the very special nature of the duty of care which exists between nurses and their patients.

The most powerful and important driver for activity in the healthcare setting, respect for personal autonomy, is explored in Chapter 6. The exercise of autonomy is unpacked in this chapter by examining empowerment, advocacy and consent in action. There are challenges in this chapter for the student and the trained nurse alike which require us to examine how we approach some of the basics of nurse–patient interaction.

Two of the most contentious issues in healthcare are examined in Chapter 7. Abortion (written by Hilary) and euthanasia (Peter) are used to explore how some of the arguments expounded elsewhere in the book might be used to generate argument, and counter-argument, in relation to ethical debate. This chapter also explores the nature of dilemmas and what these might mean for us in nursing practice. We note in this chapter how the nature of ethical debate is affected by the politics of the day.

Chapter 8, written by Hilary, places the rest of the book within the context of the realities of twenty-first-century nursing provision. It challenges nurses to take a lead in the provision of care and in doing so to act as role models for other nurses and members of the wider healthcare team. We are reminded that ethics requires us to engage with the realities of the situations before us and as such it is an important aspect of the provision of evidence-based nursing care.

Throughout the book you are provided with opportunities to think in more depth about the issues being raised. This is achieved by providing various activities for you to undertake; these activities are there to support personal and professional understanding and growth and you are encouraged to engage with them. Where an activity is very personal to you there is no specimen answer at the end of the chapter. Where we do not state there is no specimen answer, you are encouraged to look at our reflections on the activities after you have come to some conclusion for yourself.

There are case studies in the book which are drawn from real life. The case studies are used to illustrate points made within the text, to provide context to the issues being explored, as well as to allow you to reflect on what you are reading. Scenarios serve the same purpose, but they are not taken from real life rather they are our attempt to capture some of the important aspects of a discussion in a way which we hope is meaningful to the reader.

The book also uses concept summaries to highlight to you some concepts which we consider are important for you to understand. You are encouraged to engage with these summaries and perhaps use the internet or other texts to explore these further. As well as concept summaries, we have provided a glossary of some of the important and some of the difficult to understand words and short phrases in the book. Words which appear in the glossary appear in bold in the text; you are encouraged to use the glossary to ensure you get the full benefit from each chapter you read.

Finally there are issues discussed in this book which may be very pertinent to you and others and which may cause you some distress. If this is the case you are encouraged to seek the support of your mentor, personal tutor or university lecturer, who will doubtless be equipped to support you as you explore your understanding of some of the issues which occur in the day-to-day practice of nursing.

Most of all we hope this book stimulates your development as an ethically active nurse and that this ethical activity remains a feature of your entire nursing career.

Chapter 1
Introducing ethics

Peter Ellis

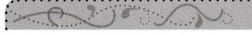

NMC Standards for Pre-registration Nursing Education

This chapter will address the following competencies:

Domain 1: Professional values

1. All nurses must practise with confidence according to *The Code: Professional Standards of Practice and Behaviour for Nurses and Midwives* (Nursing and Midwifery Council (NMC), 2015), and within other recognised ethical and legal frameworks. They must be able to recognise and address ethical challenges relating to people's choices and decision making about their care, and act within the law to help them and their families and carers find acceptable solutions.

2. All nurses must practise in a holistic, non-judgemental, caring and sensitive manner that avoids *assumptions*, supports social inclusion; recognises and respects individual choice; and acknowledges diversity. Where necessary, they must challenge inequality, discrimination and exclusion from access to care.

Domain 2: Communication and interpersonal skills

1. All nurses must build partnerships and therapeutic relationships through safe, effective and non-discriminatory communication. They must take account of individual differences, capabilities and needs.

Domain 4: Leadership, management and team working

4. All nurses must be self-aware and recognise how their own values, principles and assumptions may affect their practice. They must maintain their own personal and professional development, learning from experience, through supervision, feedback, reflection and evaluation.

NMC Essential Skills Clusters

This chapter will address the following ESCs:

Care, compassion and communication

2. People can trust the newly registered graduate nurse to engage in person-centred care empowering people to make choices about how their needs are met when they are unable to meet them for themselves.

3. People can trust the newly registered graduate nurse to respect them as individuals and strive to help them to preserve their dignity at all times.

Chapter aims

After reading this chapter you will be able to:

- discuss the practical nature of ethics;
- identify the influences which frame your own ethical beliefs;
- understand some of the values which inform ethical nursing practice;
- discuss why ethics are fundamental to good nursing practice;
- consider how ethics contribute to societal living.

Introduction

Nursing is an ethical activity. From the moment we enter the world of care and take on the mantle of student nurse we are made aware of our responsibility, not only for what we do in practice, but also, and increasingly, in our day-to-day lives outside of work. Ethical behaviour both in and outside of work contributes to the standing of the profession within society. Unethical and illegal activities bring the wider nursing profession into disrepute and will have a lasting impact on the relationships between nurses and those we care for. Simply put, good nursing relies on good relationships between nurses and patients and good relationships rely on the profession having a positive public image. The promotion and protection of the positive regard in which nurses are held in society is therefore every nurse's responsibility.

This chapter will create the backdrop for the rest of the book. While reading it you will need to be honest with yourself in exploring your personal and developing professional **values**.

Are ethics important?

Ethics as a concept means many different things to different people and, indeed, may mean something different to the same person at different stages and in different situations of that person's life. That is to say, our concept of ethics is shaped as much by our own life experiences as it is by the learning undertaken in the classroom or clinical setting.

Activity 1.1   *Reflection*

When you hear the term ethics, what word do you think of and what do these words mean to you? What do you think the term *nursing ethics* means? What words do you associate with nursing ethics and why? Write down your answers as you may wish to return to them once you have finished reading this book.

Since the answers to this activity are personal to you, there is no specimen answer at the end of the chapter.

When asked the question posed in Activity 1.1, most people say ethics is about right and wrong, good and evil, morality, philosophical questions and actions. Indeed, ethics as a concept exists in multiple dimensions; these include:

- academic/theoretical;
- personal;
- professional;
- situational;
- societal/political.

For example, academic ethics might explore some theoretical concepts of right and wrong in relation to potential new treatments, while professional ethics will examine the behaviour of individuals in their work setting. But which, if any, of these answers is correct?

In this book ethics are regarded as all of these things, but most especially as a practical undertaking which helps to guide our day-to-day activity and, more specifically for us, nursing practice. This is underlined by the NMC (2010) requirement in the *Standards for Pre-registration Nursing Education,* Domain 4: Leadership, management and team working: *All nurses must be self-aware and recognise how their own values, principles and assumptions may affect their practice.*

It is important that personal and professional ethics are compatible with each other; we cannot be caring individuals in work and callous in our day-to-day lives. One key message of this book, therefore, is the need to be attuned to our ethical self wherever we are and whatever we are doing. Sometimes this is called **ethical congruence**; in the sense used here, ethical congruence means we act in a way which is consistent and true to ourselves regardless of the situation in which we find ourselves. Jeffreys (2012) claims cultural congruence, in nursing students, is about the fit between the students' values and beliefs and those of the organisations in which they find themselves working. For organisations one might read team, ward or, at its most important, profession; so perhaps for student nurses congruence is about the fit between their personal ethical and moral values and those of the wider nursing profession into which they have entered.

Socrates, in Plato's famous book *The Republic* (translated by Lee, 1981), says ethics is no small matter because it helps us to understand *how we ought to live.* This highlights something of the nature of ethics and what ethics means. Clearly *how we ought to live* indicates ethics is about action and not about words; it is about what we do and how we behave as well as about what we think and feel – our actions as much as our expressed attitudes, if you like. Socrates' view of the purpose of ethics is that it provides guidance for us as to how we might live together in social groups, in society.

The need for an ethical code by which to live, therefore, may conceivably arise from the fact that we live in groups, communities, societies, nations and an increasingly small world. If we lived solitary lives as humans there would be very little we could do which might affect other people. The fact that what we do affects others is an important stimulus both for the existence of ethics and is a commonly held human intuition as to why we should generally behave ourselves!

Nursing takes place in a setting, be that a physical place, such as a hospital, or within a more diverse team, such as in the community. Given what we do as nurses has a direct and immediate impact on others and given those others are usually in a state of vulnerability, the need for us to understand and adhere to a code of ethical behaviour becomes more apparent.

Activity 1.2 invites you to consider the far-reaching nature of ethics and its implications for our place in the world in general. It is important to remember that what we do as human beings does not take place in a vacuum; what we do has an impact on someone, somewhere, at some time.

Activity 1.2   *Reflection*

Consider some important modern ethical issues. What are the features of the issues which make them ethical, about right and wrong, rather than just mundane problems? If you are struggling, think about global warming, for example: what is it that makes this an ethical rather than, say, merely a practical, scientific or climatic problem?

There are some possible answers to all activities at the end of the chapter, unless otherwise indicated.

The important thing about ethics is the way in which they guide us in our relationships with others. Ethics help us consider questions such as, 'what is the right thing to do?' and 'what are the consequences of this action?' What should be clear from your answer to Activity 1.2 is that ethical questions refer to the right thing to do and the consequences of our actions in relation to how they affect other people. Of course such arguments operate not only at the human level but also at a professional level, where the basis for ethical behaviour is more formal (see Chapter 8). The distinction between *doing the right thing* and doing something to ensure *the right outcome* is an important one (see Chapter 4).

One seventeenth-century philosopher, Thomas Hobbes, described a theory of 'natural rights', which adds a further dimension to our understanding of why ethics (of which **rights** are one branch; see Chapter 5) are so important (Hobbes, edited by Tuck, 1991). For Hobbes, the one natural right for humans was the *right to self-preservation*. Before we lived in societies humans survived in any way they could. According to Hobbes, life in this *natural state* was *short, uncomfortable and quite brutal.* Because of the severe nature of life in the *natural state* humans moved to living in communities to gain an increasing level of comfort and longevity of life (Hobbes, edited by Tuck, 1991).

To achieve self-preservation and to improve our lives, Hobbes believed we needed a social contract (an implicit agreement) which respected our individual and collective right to self-preservation. What we can take from this idea is something quite simple, but at the same time quite profound: ethics makes our collective and individual lives better. Hobbes' 'natural rights' reflect a good understanding of what we consider to be basic **human rights** now; for example, the **right to life**, the right to safety from violence. What is most important about any notion of ethics and human rights is they do, and must, apply to everyone in equal measure. It is this notion that rights belong to everyone which often causes us concern when we see the how some regimes treat their citizens, even though what we see has no direct impact on us.

The idea of achieving a better life for everyone resounds throughout the history of ethics and ethical theories: notably Aristotle (translated by Thompson, 1976) describes 'the good life' as one in which people both do well and live well; they achieve their potential and do so ethically. Sometimes this is called **human flourishing** – that is doing, being and feeling well and achieving one's potential. What is increasingly clear here is that the understanding of why ethics is important has clear parallels with why nursing is important (to make people's lives more comfortable and help them attain their goals) as well as with how nurses should follow a code of conduct; as nurses we are therefore exhorted to both live and nurse well!

This concept of ethics is therefore about a mutually observed contract in which all parties abide by certain standards of behaviour both for their own benefit as well as for the benefit of others. It is on the occasions when this contract breaks down that life returns to Hobbes' *short, uncomfortable and brutal state* in which no one really benefits. Activity 1.3 points to a fictitious example of this, although, regrettably, there are many similar real-life examples.

Activity 1.3 — *Reflection*

Go online and find a synopsis of the book *Lord of the Flies* by William Golding. Consider the nature of the story in relation to societal norms, ethical behaviour and the potential consequences of life without ethical guidance.

If you undertake Activity 1.3, and also perhaps reflect on periods in history when ethical norms have been abandoned, you will identify some of the consequences of the failure to live by the 'social contract'. Living by a code of conduct in society at large makes life worth living for humans in general. Obviously the argument being made here is not to suggest notions of ethics and ethical principles led to the formation of society as such, but that once humans started to live in groups the practicalities of societal living required some rules by which we should live.

It is no surprise that the ethical code by which we live as human beings in general is not as well defined or laid out as the code of conduct for nursing. The power of the ethical code of conduct for nurses comes not only from the fact we are humans, but also as a result of the fact that on entering the nursing profession we choose to submit ourselves to additional rules. These rules which we accept as nurses are part of a contract we have with society. We live by the rules and therefore people know what to expect of us when they interact with nurses and nurses are given a level of respect by the general public as a result, as well as being paid to do the work of caring (for a clearer explanation of the notion of **special rights** and **special responsibilities**, see Chapter 5).

We have seen that everyone has a need to abide by some form of ethics in order for society to function. But ethics exist and operate at many more levels than this. For example, when someone takes on any job, that person enters into a contract of employment which is both explicit (in that it is written down and therefore both ethical and legal) and implicit (i.e. an employer can expect certain behaviours). A good example is the standard of reasonable and polite behaviour we might expect in a restaurant or supermarket. Such behaviour is a requirement of employment and for student nurses can be found in both the university code of student discipline and the NHS contract – this is an example of a special (ethical as well as legal) responsibility.

People take on a further layer of ethical responsibility when entering a profession. This responsibility is laid out in the professional code of conduct for that profession. Such codes arise as a result of the extra faith individuals place in professionals who they turn to at particular times of their lives. Professionals are rewarded for belonging to and operating as a professional in whatever setting. Professionals have a status in society, are paid (usually better than the norm) and are allowed freedoms within their professional lives which are not given to others (for example, prescribing and administering medications). Because such rights place the professional in a position of **power**, as well as because in some situations these rights are open to abuse, codes of conduct serve as an extra layer of protection for the client. Codes of conduct identify what the professional is and isn't allowed to do and provide guidance for professionals in managing their relationship with clients. In this way codes of conduct, like contracts of employment, reflect the notion of the social contract discussed earlier, except they are much more specific in relating to certain jobs and professional roles.

Nursing, as a profession, requires us to intervene in people's lives at a point when they need a lot of support and may be vulnerable. In these situations *The Code* serves as a means of protecting the **interests** of the patient or client and as nurses we accept the rules as part and parcel of how we ought to act; they are a more specific form of social contract if you like – the nursing code of conduct does not apply to people who are not nurses, midwives or health visitors (or students of these professions).

Activity 1.4   *Critical thinking*

Go online to the NMC website and find a copy of

The Code: Professional Standards of Practice and Behaviour for Nurses and Midwives. Look at the section entitled 'Promote professionalism and trust' and reflect on what this means in relation to the messages in this chapter so far.

Since the answers to this activity are personal to you, there is no specimen answer at the end of the chapter.

The Code (NMC, 2015) highlights how the conduct of nurses, midwives and health visitors relates to the wider public and public perception of our professions in that it exhorts us to:

- prioritise people;
- practise effectively;

- preserve safety;
- promote professionalism and trust.

What we see is reference to 'people' and 'trust', the reference is not just to patients (it does not say prioritise patients), as well as the need to maintain trust in the profession. The choice of wording here supports the argument made thus far: ethics are important for life in general and not something we can choose to switch on only when we are at work.

Understanding values

So far we have identified that ethics are an important aspect of life in society and life without ethical codes might prove challenging and potentially dangerous. The questions that arise for us as nurses are:

- What do ethics require of us?
- What values should guide our ethical thinking and behaviours?

The contract which we enter into on joining the nursing profession is reflected in some of the standards of proficiency from the NMC. Take, for example, Domain 1: Professional values 2, where the NMC states:

> *All nurses must practise in a holistic, non-judgemental, caring and sensitive manner that avoids assumptions, supports social inclusion; recognises and respects individual choice; and acknowledges diversity. Where necessary, they must challenge inequality, discrimination and exclusion from access to care.*

The clear message here is not about passive acceptance of rules and 'doing the right thing', but about standing up for others where necessary – that is prioritising people. The requirement on nursing, and indeed all health and social care professions, includes going out of our way to do good and protect and promote the wellbeing of others. In part this standing up for others might manifest itself as the act of **advocacy** (discussed in Chapter 6) and at other times this may require something more, such as challenging poor or dangerous practice as well as policy and planning which might be inequitable.

Furthermore, Domain 4: Leadership, management and team working 4, points to interesting requirements for nursing practice in that nurses need to be:

> *self-aware and recognise how their own values, principles and assumptions may affect their practice. They must maintain their own personal and professional development, learning from experience, through supervision, feedback, reflection and evaluation.*

This points to an interesting and important message – all nurses are different. There may seem to be a tension here between the aim of having all nurses work in accordance with *The Code* and expressly recognising they too have their own values. This tension only arises if our own values are at odds with those of the profession to which we belong, as it is our values, principles and assumptions which guide our individual behaviours. To understand this better, as well as to meet the challenge of the NMC proficiencies, we must first understand what values are and then identify and understand our own values.

What then are values? Most notably Schwartz (1992) describes values as being beliefs which relate to a desirable outcome of a given behaviour; values are more important than individual situations, allowing us to choose between, or appraise, behaviours or outcomes. Schwartz suggests we order values according to what we consider to be important and these values motivate us in what we do and how we behave both individually and in groups. For Schwartz (1994), values are a response to three *universal requirements*:

1.   the needs of humans as biological organisms;
2.   requisites of coordinated social interaction;
3.   the smooth working and survival of groups.

Schwartz (1994) identifies ten values:

1. security;
2. conformity;
3. tradition;
4. benevolence;
5. universalism;
6. self-direction;
7. stimulation;
8. hedonism;
9. achievement;
10. power.

What these mean in practice is not always obvious. But if we take benevolence as an example, how this is displayed and the meaning it has for the individual and for others includes being honest, being helpful, being loyal, taking responsibility and valuing friendship. As nurses, clearly benevolence is something we should all value highly.

Essentially the actions which underpin values are driven by attitudes and beliefs which we cherish as human beings (Jiga-Boy et al., 2016). Such beliefs are so important to us that they are not altered by situations in which we find ourselves (so if we were starving we might feel bad about stealing a loaf of bread, even if we did so to stay alive or to feed our children). The beliefs which we have as individuals are often shared by people who are like us and so act like we do. We therefore admire the actions of such individuals as their actions are seen as displaying our shared values and beliefs; conversely, we are wary of, or even despise, people who act in ways which are contrary to our values.

People who enter the caring professions usually share common values and beliefs and expect these to be displayed by other people in similar caring roles. As a society we tend to admire people who demonstrate these values in the way they interact and care for others. Some students find it hard to adapt to some of the values of more seasoned professionals, or fail to understand the values which motivate them. Understanding the values which motivate you as a nurse is important. Values can provide a point of reference when we confront difficult ethical situations. Activity 1.5 asks you to identify some of your own values as well as those of some of the people you work with. Understanding and responding to your own values will help motivate you and will highlight to you when things are not as they should be in the practice setting.

Activity 1.5   *Critical thinking*

Consider the reasons which brought you into nursing. What values underpin what you try to achieve as a nurse? As well as identifying the values, write a sentence about what each value means and how you might show it in action. You may like to write them down and perhaps discuss them with colleagues, your mentor or tutor. Look for the similarities and differences between your answers and think about why this might be.

Activity 1.5 asks you to identify your own values. Knowing, understanding and living according to your values has a number of advantages:

- It sets a clear pattern for how you should behave and enables you to avoid acting in ways you might regret later.
- It enhances your ability to make what are good decisions about things quickly, coherently and consistently.
- You will be able to prioritise what you want from life and how you will achieve it.
- It helps you to find your own identity and readily identify people like you who you want to have as friends and colleagues.
- It enables you to be true to yourself and live a life that makes sense; it enhances integrity.
- If you live by your values people will learn to trust you.

The argument being made thus far suggests therefore that your priorities and values as a person should be the same as those you have as a nurse; indeed it would prove difficult to live according to one set of values as a nurse and another set in your private life. Try Activity 1.6.

Activity 1.6   *Reflection*

Make a list of the things which are important to you as a person. Use single words where possible, so where you might write 'being the best I can be', instead put 'achievement'. Now take your answers to Activity 1.5, and again turn your answers into single words, so 'to care for people' becomes just 'caring'. Lastly compare the two lists. Look for words which might have a similar basis, such as 'love' and 'care'. Now reflect on whether the two lists actually contain similar ideas. What do these lists say about you both as a nurse and as a person?

Where there is a mismatch between a person's values and behaviours as a nurse and his or her personal values and behaviours, stress and tension will result. Nurses who only pretend to value human life in work but who out of work do not live by the same values will inevitably start to demonstrate the incongruence in the workplace – they will be short-tempered, perhaps harsh with patients and show apathy where they should show concern. It is at this point that patient care will become affected and the individual's integrity and fitness to be a nurse will be called into question.

Professional and personal values are largely inseparable from each other. Our value systems and beliefs shape the ways in which we think, feel and behave. Our values shape our personal identity – the person we present to the world at large. We said at the start of this chapter that ethics is about informing not only what we think and feel but also our actions. Within the sphere of professional life the way in which we behave towards others shapes our professional identity and indeed the identity we choose has an impact on how we behave. It is worth thinking about how professional identities are developed and what impact they have on us as we develop our professional persona.

Professional identities

One of the outcomes of nurse education is the socialisation of nursing students to the values and behaviours of nursing in general. Think of it like this at its most stark: when young student nurses start nursing they may have just left school, they may have limited life experience and may not know *how* they will act and react to various events. In their role as a student nurse they are confronted with behaviours and scenarios which are outside their sphere of experience to date, so how do they know how to react? How do they cope with some of the more challenging, and potentially frightening, scenarios? Nursing education aims to help students to adapt and learn to cope with these scenarios while displaying the right behaviours and values. The example set by their mentors and other staff in the practice setting also contributes to this adaptation and evolution of students' identity.

It is not always easy to know how a student's professional identity might develop. This lack of clarity is perhaps as true of older students who come with more life, and possibly care, experience as it is of younger students. Clearly the greatest influences on the behaviours and understanding of students are the actions and explanations they see and hear from more experienced people around them – this may include other, perhaps older or more practised, nursing students. These actions and explanations are processed and reflected upon by inexperienced nurses who have to decide whether to accept or reject them, to add them to their values and ways of behaving or not. This process of developing one's own identity within the context of a new culture is often described in the nursing literature as **acculturation** (Brown et al., 2012). In the sense used here acculturation refers to the developing understanding and adopting of the culture of nursing by the student nurse. It is by adopting the culture, and **cultural norms** of nursing that the student moves from being an outsider to 'one of us', a nurse, one of the culture.

What is happening here is the student is creating new understandings about behaviours and attitudes; these attitudes and behaviours may be adopted by students and form part of their emerging professional identity (Blais and Hayes, 2015). Socialisation into nursing norms of behaviour and values takes place more in the practice setting than in the classroom; remember we said earlier that ethics is as much a practical pursuit as an academic one. It is here, at the cutting edge of nursing, that identities are created. Our identity as humans results from reflection on our experiences and observations about things we have seen and been involved with; our identity as nurses is shaped, for better or for worse, in the same way through reflection on our practice experience.

Of course, one of the dangers of learning through observation of others is the behaviours and displayed attitudes of others who may themselves be flawed, or we may choose to reject what are reasonable behaviours and attitudes. Often nursing students report behaviours in practice, by other nurses, which they find upsetting or which they know are wrong. These issues create a clear message for us when thinking about the creation of personal values, ethics and identities from the start of our nursing lives: we need to be mindful of what sort of nurse, and indeed person, we choose to become.

When examining *The Code* (NMC, 2015) you were asked to consider the section entitled 'Promote professionalism and trust'. If we were to look at the other three key statement areas we would see how collectively they provide a basis for the values we need to function ethically and professionally as nurses in the twenty-first century. The key statements are to:

* prioritise people;
* practise effectively;
* preserve safety.

Respecting individuals

One of the fundamental aspects of ethical life, and nursing ethics in particular, is the need to avoid judging people. *The Code* (NMC, 2015, p 15) requires nurses to:

stay objective and have clear professional boundaries at all times with people in your care (including those who have been in your care in the past), their families and carers.

Clearly there are a number of issues with such a position and many challenges for nurses who have to care for people who, in the ordinary course of events, they may not choose to have anything to do with. There are also personal ethical and moral issues which may arise from our individual moral and religious viewpoints.

A good way to pull this idea into focus alongside the notion of personal and professional identity is to consider the notion of **binary thinking**.

Theory summary: binary thinking

One of the ways we can generate an identity for ourselves is to compare certain characteristics of ours with those of other people. For example, I am a man, you may be a woman; I am a lecturer, you may be a student; I am a nurse, you are a patient. The point here is that identity is defined

(continued)

(continued)

by difference – a process sometimes called **othering** (Davies, 2003). We create a social identity for ourselves which sets us apart from people who are 'not like us'. Of course, in the process of creating a professional identity this may be a positive as we strive to become more caring than the norm, say, but equally this idea may be detrimental as we use difference to create a bubble around our collective identity as nurses and perhaps choose not to allow *others* into our group.

Where this takes us on our ethical journey is to a point where we need to think clearly and rationally about the values that drive us, the identities these create and what this means for our interactions with others.

One of the defining features of the professional identity has always been the knowledge which professions have. It is the possession of this knowledge and the skills and means to exercise this knowledge which generates the difference between persons within the profession and those from outside (the other). So, for example, we might consider the classic, although admittedly stereotyped, notion of the all-knowing surgeon and the grateful, ignorant patient. Of course as nurses we possess a body of knowledge and we have access to the skills and the tools to use this knowledge. We may choose therefore to create an identity for ourselves in which we take the view that we are the professional and we know what is in the patient's (the other's) **best interests** – that is, we choose to become the 'all-knowing' nurse. Conversely we can choose a different identity for ourselves, one in which we work in partnership with people to make sure [we] deliver care effectively (NMC, 2015, p. 4) and apply our knowledge and skills alongside our patients', recognising the things we have in common (our humanity, our cares, our fears).

The suggestion here is that by dwelling on our differences – what sets us apart from (or perhaps what we might consider makes us better than) other people – we generate artificial barriers, a sort of *them and us*, if you like, and this stands in the way of both useful and ethical relationships with patients (and indeed our peers). These barriers are created to support things which are perhaps not **morally relevant** (they have no ethical worth) when what we should be concentrating on is our common humanity and issues of identity which have some moral meaning. But how is this achieved?

Activity 1.7   *Decision making*

At this point it is worth making some decisions about what sort of person makes a good nurse. We have seen that one way of creating an identity for ourselves is to choose characteristics which show us as separate from others. Think about the notion of binary identity and othering and decide for yourself what sort of characteristics you might adopt to help make you the sort of person and nurse described in the NMC Standards and associated Essential Skills Clusters identified at the start of this chapter.

In the NMC Essential Skills Clusters, skill 3 in the domain of 'Care, compassion and communication' states:

People can trust the newly registered graduate nurse to respect them as individuals and strive to help them the preserve their dignity at all times.

Respecting individuals and preserving their dignity might be hard to achieve if we choose an identity based on notions of difference at best and superiority at worst. Where the challenge lies for us as nurses is to construct for ourselves a set of values which include respect for others and which are more powerful than any notion of professional identity. Values such as respect for dignity and humanity should not just be values we give lip service to but should be demonstrated in *who we are* and how we behave towards others.

It is difficult to put into words exactly what this means. But if we consider what we would like in the way of behaviour from others if we, or a loved one, were to be a consumer of care we may start to get somewhere close to understanding what respect, dignity and humanity might look like in action. So if we value other people as equals, then we may be described as respectful; if we value the dignity of others we may be described as noble; and if we display humanity we can claim compassion as a facet of our professional identity.

Case study: showing respect for humanity

Edith Cavell was a British nurse who lived and worked in Belgium. Throughout her short nursing service in the First World War, Edith helped the wounded from either side without any discrimination. She clearly chose to consider the moral elements of her calling to be a nurse and care for the sick and injured. Sadly she was executed in 1915 for helping Allied soldiers escape occupied Belgium. Edith Cavell clearly displayed the ability to put the welfare of others before her professional, or indeed national, identity. You can find a statue in her honour at St Martin's Place in the northeast corner of Trafalgar Square, London.

Of course the courage which Edith Cavell showed is not something which many of us will ever need to draw on in our professional lives. Her ability to care for other people, regardless of whether or not they were the enemy, demonstrates the moral benchmark which we have as nurses: respecting individuals for their humanity; respecting characteristics which are *morally relevant.*

In Chapter 3 we start to look at ideas of what ethics is and what ethics is not, which will add further to our understanding of some of the ideas contained in this chapter. For now though, we will consider: do values, personal and professional identity and respecting others help us to make our lives, and the lives of those around us, better?

Is ethics a nursing concern?

One of the key features of nursing ethics which distinguishes it from ethics per se, and medical ethics in particular, is the emphasis nursing ethics places on care, rather than cure. This emphasis on care reflects strongly the belief of most nurses, and nurse theorists, that the relationship with the individual patient, is as important as, if not more important than, what is actually done for and with the patient. This may seem like an odd thing to say but there are a number of reasons why this is the starting point for ethical nursing practice.

So why is our relationship to our patients at least as important ethically as what we do? First, and as we shall see in Chapter 4, one of the important features of ethical and moral behaviour is the **intent** which underlies it. Intent is the stimulus for how we act and why we choose to do what we do. What is important about intent is that sometimes the outcome of an action is not what we primarily intended it to be, but because we acted from the right motives, or with the right intent, the action is nevertheless regarded as ethical.

The notion of the relationship in care being at least as important as cure is further thrown into stark relief when we consider the content of many of the complaints received by the National Health Service (NHS) each year. NHS Digital (2014) reported that 21.6 per cent of all complaints received about the NHS in the year 2012–2013 were about staff attitude and poor communication. If ethics is about attitudes and values and these attitudes and values drive behaviours, such as how we choose to communicate with others, then clearly there remains some work to be done in the caring professions.

Case study: showing disrespect for humanity

In April 2014 a BBC documentary uncovered a regime of physical and emotional abuse at the Old Deanery care home in Essex. Staff at the home, who were supposed to care for elderly people, some with dementia and others who were terminally ill, were slapping, mocking and ignoring residents' calls for help.

What this case study shows is that even in a caring environment it is easy for people, who may previously have been caring individuals, to allow themselves to start regarding those they look after as *other* at best and perhaps merely as objects at worst. When respect for people is lost then bad things happen, and in nursing that often means to the most vulnerable in society. Working ethically is therefore a nursing concern.

If we were to explore further the concept of caring as fundamental to nursing ethics and nursing practice, we might examine the focus of any of the models of nursing. They point us to actions which are intended to support patients in:

- their activities of daily living (Roper et al., 1980);
- achieving self-care (Orem, 1991);
- adapting (Roy and Andrews, 1999).

These models do not point to cure as an aspect of nursing; instead they indicate a preoccupation with the *human*, or humane, aspects of care, the sorts of things which are important for human beings. You might remember toward the start of the chapter we identified Socrates and Aristotle as describing ethics as a means of living together in social groups (supporting, or at least allowing, people to fulfil the activities of daily living) as well as society providing one means to achieving the *good life* through reaching our potential, *flourishing* (achieving self-care and adapting) ethically.

So is ethics a nursing concern? Of course it is! We live and work in society. Not only that, we live and work among some of the most vulnerable people in society and in order to assist others to reach their own full potential we, as nurses, need to act in a manner which is both ethical and enabling. As the case study above shows, this may mean intervening to stop the spread of systematic abuse.

All of the above looks quite onerous – hard to achieve and to live by. What should be apparent, however, to any student is that an individual does not become a nurse overnight; as with all facets of care, nurses progressively take on more responsibility, gain more understanding and socialise into the role. Henderson, a prominent and still very influential nursing theorist, said in 1966:

> *Every nurse has to develop her own concept [of morality], otherwise she is merely imitating others or acting under authority.*

What Henderson is saying here, and the important message for this chapter, is that nurses need both to have and to enact their own moral code, otherwise they become mere puppets acting in ways in which others see fit. This can lead to nurses acting in ways which are in contrast to the express aims of nursing. When a nurse acts in a manner which is at odds with the values which s/he holds this can lead to **moral stress**. Lützén et al. (2003), in their synthesis of data from two qualitative studies, show that moral stress in nursing is generated because:

- nurses are morally sensitive to the vulnerability of patients;
- external pressures often prevent nurses from acting in ways which they consider to be in patients' best interests;
- nurses therefore feel out of control.

The argument in this chapter so far is that ethics is good for society in general and the exercise of ethics is good for the wellbeing of people and nurses in particular. Being sensitive to the vulnerabilities of others is clearly a good thing and is one of the characteristics which defines good nursing, but how do we then cope when lack of resources or conflicts of professional power mean we are pressurised to act in a manner which we regard as not being proper and, more importantly, morally right?

Wainwright (1991, p. 46) suggests:

> *What qualifies someone to speak on ethical matters, in the context of professional practice, is not so much their knowledge of the profession (although this may be important) as their understanding of moral philosophy.*

Of course this is a little idealised, but the suggestion here is that understanding and being able to argue clearly and in an ethically informed way are important steps in being able to influence moral and ethical decision making. So the suggestion is, at least in part, that it is a requirement nurses learn and understand something of the nature, language and practice of ethics.

It might further be argued that an increased understanding of ethics and ethical decision making and activity in nursing might usefully contribute to the collective professional identity of nursing, which we discussed earlier.

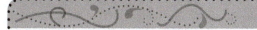

Chapter summary

This chapter has provided a quick overview of what we mean by ethics and the reasons why ethics is important in society at large, for patient care and for nursing and individual nurses in particular. We have identified what values are and how these might be used to shape the ways in which we act in both our private and our professional lives.

We identified nursing as having a specific professional identity of which we need to be aware in order that we avoid imposing that identity in a way which constrains others. As a counterbalance to this we identified that respect for individuals should be a cornerstone of ethical nursing practice.

We noted that ethics and morality are the business of every nurse and that a grasp of the language, nature and activity of ethics is an important first step in helping us come to grips with the often morally stressful nature of care provision.

Activities: brief outline answers

Activity 1.2 Reflection

What the big ethical questions have in common is that the consequences of certain actions, and indeed the actions themselves, all relate to human life. Global warming may impoverish lives and reduce life expectancy both now and in the future; of course there are arguments about what we are doing to the planet in general, but many of these revolve around the impact on current and future generations. Not providing social care will impact on the lives of the elderly, infirm and the poor – not to mention the dehumanising effect this has on societies in general. Migration affects the lives of the people entering the UK, some to escape persecution and violence, but it also affects the lives of people already living in the UK, perhaps relating to increased demand on resources. Questions about **abortion** affect potential mothers, potential babies and societal conscience in general. Higher speed limits may allow people to get around quicker but may endanger life – which is more important therefore?

Activity 1.3 Reflection

What we see in this book is the stranded boys drifting towards something resembling Hobbes' natural state where there is lawlessness and a lack of ethical and moral behaviour. As a result life becomes brutish and short for some. This, albeit fictional, account of life without rules demonstrates something of the argument being made here: ethical rules and social and cultural norms and boundaries exist to make our lives better and less brutish.

Activity 1.5 Critical thinking

Answers to this question will almost certainly include: 'to care for people', 'to make a difference', 'to improve people's lives'. These answers point to the fact that people are important to nurses and people come in all shapes, sizes, colours, classes and with all manner of belief systems and behaviours. What is relevant to nurses is simply this: patients are people and people deserve our care. Of course we may have other values in our lives, like respect for other people's freedoms and choices; again, these reflect some of the proficiencies the NMC requires from us as nurses.

Activity 1.6 Reflection

For many of you there are areas of great similarity between the two value lists you have created. For you there is something inevitable about your choice of nursing as a career as it fulfils a need to express your values through what you do. For some there will be areas of tension between the values on one list and the other; these tensions, if not too large, are probably normal as you enter a career in nursing. They are something to be aware of and think about as you socialise into your new identity. Where there are areas of major conflict between what you value as a person and what you value as a nurse, you will need to think hard about how you might address these.

Activity 1.7 Decision making

In this chapter you have already been challenged to think about the values which may be associated with being a good nurse. This activity is a further challenge, asking you to decide how you will behave in relation to others in the construction of your own identity. One way to avoid the pitfalls of binary thinking is to construct an identity around the things which make us similar as human beings rather than what makes us different. So perhaps defining yourself as a person first is a good place to start. Caring, respectful and autonomous might be further themes worth developing, especially where we value these things in, and for, others as much as we do for ourselves.

Further reading

Davies, C (2003) Workers, professions and identity, in Henderson, J and Atkinson, D (eds) *Managing Care in Context*. London: Routledge.

de Araujo Sartorio, N and Lourdes Campos Pavone Zoboli, E (2010) Images of a 'good nurse' presented by teaching staff. *Nursing Ethics*, 17(6): 687–694.
A thought-provoking study into what nurse teachers in Brazil consider to be a good nurse.

Engward, H (2010) Exploring undergraduate student nurses' situated experiences of ethics: centring students through story discussions. *Occasional Papers in Education and Lifelong Learning: An International Journal*, 4(1–2): 49–62.
A useful study into how undergraduate students view ethics.

Mooney, M (2007) Professional socialization: the key to survival as a newly qualified nurse. *International Journal of Nursing Practice*, 13: 75–80.
A good insight into the process of socialising into the nursing profession.

Winters, N (2016) Seeking status: the process of becoming and remaining an emergency nurse. *Journal of Emergency Nursing*, 42(5): 412–419.
An interesting insight into the socialisation of nurses in the emergency department.

Useful websites

www.bbc.co.uk/news/uk-england-bristol-20078999
A chronological view of the abuse scandal at Winterbourne View care home.

www.icn.ch/who-we-are/code-of-ethics-for-nurses
The International Council of Nurses' code of ethics can be found here.

www.nmc-uk.org
The online presence of the Nursing and Midwifery Council, where relevant publications, such as *The Code*, can be found.

www.mindtools.com/pages/article/newTED_85.htm
An interesting take on what values are and how you might identify yours.

Chapter 2
Using reflection to develop inductive ethical understanding

Lioba Howatson-Jones and Peter Ellis

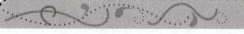

NMC Standards for Pre-registration Nursing Education

This chapter will address the following competencies:

Domain 1: Professional values

1. All nurses must practise with confidence according to *The Code: Professional Standards of Practice and Behaviour for Nurses and Midwives* (NMC, 2015), and within other recognised ethical and legal frameworks. They must be able to recognise and address ethical challenges relating to people's choices and decision making about their care, and act within the law to help them and their families and carers find acceptable solutions.

Domain 2: Communication and interpersonal skills

8. All nurses must respect individual rights to confidentiality and keep information secure and confidential in accordance with the law and relevant ethical and regulatory frameworks, taking account of local protocols. They must also actively share personal information with others when the interests of safety and protection override the need for confidentiality.

NMC Essential Skills Clusters

This chapter will address the following ESCs:

Care, compassion and communication

1. As partners in the care process, people can trust a newly registered graduate nurse to provide collaborative care based on the highest standards, knowledge and competence.

By the first progression point:

1. Articulates the underpinning values of *The Code: Professional Standards of Practice and Behaviour for Nurses and Midwives* (NMC, 2015).

(continued)

continued . . .

By the second progression point:

6. Forms appropriate and constructive professional relationships with families and other carers.

Cluster: Organisational aspects of care

12. People can trust the newly registered graduate nurse to respond to their feedback and a wide range of other sources to learn, develop and improve services.

By the first progression point:

1. Responds appropriately to compliments and comments.

By the second progression point:

3. Uses supervision and other forms of reflective learning to make effective use of feedback.

Chapter aims

After reading the chapter you should be able to:

*   understand how ethical values develop and become embedded through reflective practice;
*   describe how reflexive responses contribute to ethical decision making;
*   collaborate in critically reflective ethical problem solving;
*   justify how an **inductive** approach to ethical decision making is important.

Introduction

Some theoretical introduction to ethics is needed to prime the development of the ethically active nurse. This chapter builds on this foundation and the examination of your own values suggested in Chapter 1 by encouraging you to continue to develop a **practice-grounded** understanding (that is, an understanding which is based on the realities of care work and your experience of it) of ethics and ethical nursing activity through the use of reflection in and on action.

As Manu's reflection below suggests, acting ethically and in congruence with your values can be a challenging endeavour and not one which is purely confined to the practice situation. This chapter will particularly focus on how reflection and reflexivity contribute to the development of ethical values and how their use influences how these values become embedded in what we do and who we are. We are not suggesting reflection and reflexivity contribute to the development of values and understanding overnight; these insights emerge over time through reflection and reflexive responses to practice situations and collaborative learning among other ways of learning.

This chapter will also examine how the development of ethical thinking and behaviours underpinned by reflection on and in action allows the nurse to develop an inductive approach to ethical decision making. That is to say, the development of self as a reflective practitioner allows us to develop the skills necessary to employ ethical thinking strategies to help us make decisions about how and why to act rather than using ethical theory and understanding as a way of justifying what we have done. This notion of using ethical thinking to guide our actions rather than using them to justify what we have done is an important feature of this book as we regard ethical understanding to be a tool to be used to influence behaviours in practice.

Case study: Manu's values in action

Manu had come into nursing because she wanted to make a difference to people's lives. She particularly enjoyed working with people with learning disabilities because she found them interesting to talk to and she felt their way of being always challenged her to think differently about things. Manu had a hectic life outside of work with three children and elderly parents to care for. She often found herself juggling work and home life.

On this particular day she was doing the weekly shop for her parents. As she was queuing to pay, she overheard the checkout assistant talking in derogatory terms to a colleague on the other till about a customer. The store manager was also drawn into this conversation. When Manu arrived at the till the conversation continued as if she was not there.

Manu had a moment's reflection on whether to say something as she packed her bags. She decided that she could not let this go unchallenged. In as polite a tone as possible Manu asked the checkout assistant if she thought it was appropriate to talk about a customer in this way. The checkout assistant responded that it was none of Manu's business. Manu calmly replied that talking about a customer in the public area made it her business. The manager came to see what the fuss was about. Manu outlined her reasons for challenging this conversation: people have problems in their lives which are unknown, making derogatory judgements reflected badly on the store reputation and customer care focusing on her needs at the checkout was missing.

*In view of this reasoned argument the store manager had to agree that Manu was right to have challenged this discourteous behaviour and apologised. When Manu got to her parents' home she reflected briefly on what had occurred while putting the shopping away. She felt the contrast between her values of **person-centredness** and those of the store staff, who she imagined viewed people as objects. She saw that other people had been agitated by the words used, but had not responded, thereby seeming to condone the behaviour of the checkout assistant. Manu had felt impelled to challenge the checkout assistant because her innate values did not allow her to behave differently in her private life to how she would behave had she been in her work uniform, and therefore recognisable as a nurse.*

As Manu reflected further, she imagined the checkout assistant might have reacted differently to her challenge had she been in uniform because it could have exerted positional power. However, Manu

(continued)

continued . . .

> *questioned the need for exerting such power. Manu saw that this could also be an issue in practice where she tried to work ethically, but nevertheless her service users might feel pressurised to respond in ways she deemed to be acceptable. From this thinking Manu saw the need to continue to use reflection to examine her ethical intent in all situations in order to derive learning she could apply to her practice and way of being in the world.*

What this scenario points out, and what forms the backbone of this chapter, are two key important interrelated issues. The first is that Manu knew what she had to do because she was fully aware of what sort of person she is, what she values and what she finds acceptable – she reflected in action. She has arrived at this understanding through reflection on various scenarios throughout her career – perhaps an extended example of reflection on previous actions. Second, and importantly, Manu took the opportunity to reflect on what she had done, reflection on action. This allowed her to confirm to herself that what she had done was right; but more importantly, this reflection on action allowed her to confirm to herself that this was the way in which she would continue to act in the future.

Developing ethical values through reflection

Taft and White (2007) make the point that it is through reflection students begin to integrate their personal ethical beliefs with ways of being in the world which are real and meaningful, rather than developing knowledge of abstract ideas which are not truly lived values. What this means is students are able to attach what they know and what they feel to some concrete examples upon which they are able to reflect and therefore both learn from as well as come to some understanding of how they will behave in future similar situations. This is important as it demonstrates both the necessity and value of reflection for embedding positive values and associated ethical behaviours into who we are. In this way not only do we learn from experience, but we grow and develop as people by reflecting on it.

Reflection is used, employing different orientations focusing on technical issues to improve practice; deliberation to consider the alternatives available; **dialectically** (which questions wider issues such as political, social and ethical systems or the use of power) or the **transpersonal**, which focuses on personal development (Wellington and Austin, 1996).

Reflection, therefore, will also vary in depth and outcome. For the purposes of this book the latter two are of greatest relevance because they focus on issues through developing awareness and questions about the political and social systems (and the provision of care takes place within social systems) in which they exist; they also look at how individuals integrate their inner self with the self which they present to others. This transpersonal reflection is of special importance to nurses (as indeed it is in the scenario earlier which featured Manu), as it is through personal development we become the nurse we wish to be.

The notion of congruence between the inner self and the self presented to others is important in the development of self as an ethical being – as discussed in Chapter 1. One of the big challenges which faces student nurses is the development of a persona which is true to both who you are as a person and who you are as a nurse.

What we know about ourselves and the way we think and act can be reflected upon. Less obvious are the aspects of ourselves that we are not aware of, but which nevertheless infiltrate our thinking and actions. Reflecting on what might be hidden from our awareness is an important part of the inductive process. For example, we may think that we are fair and inclusive without realising that because we have a particular view of what is fair that we also have a view as to what is unfair – entrenched views such as this may lead us to form negative opinions of other people whom we see as acting in ways which we regard as being unfair. That is to say our own, unchallenged values and opinions can lead us to make judgements about others which are perhaps based on weak tenets and which are therefore of themselves unfair.

Knowing ourselves and developing a self-awareness which leads us constantly to question and refine our values, opinions and understandings are therefore important elements in the development of real ethical understanding. It is therefore important at this stage to consider how we understand ourselves before trying to make sense of the world around us. Complete Activity 2.1 to help you develop real self-awareness of your values and an understanding of how you view the world.

Activity 2.1   *Critical reflection*

The Johari window was created to help raise self-awareness about public and hidden areas of awareness within human interactions (Luft and Ingham, 1955). The Johari window is essentially a square window split into four panes; each of these panes represents a different view of the characteristics of an individual, either from that person's own view or from the view of others. The panes ask:

- What do we and others know about ourselves?
- What do others know about us which we may not be aware of?
- What is hidden from ourselves and others?
- What do we know about ourselves, but keep hidden from others?

Through a process of introspection and reflection, consider what you know about your-self within the above areas and how you can seek feedback from others to assist your self-awareness. You may find it useful to go online and read about the Johari window; a link to a webpage about the Johari window is provided at the end of the chapter.

As this is based on your own experience there is no outline answer at the end of the chapter.

What Activity 2.1 points out to us is that there is more than one way of viewing who we are and what we are about. It challenges us as individuals to consider not only what we know about who we are and what we value, but also how we represent this to the world. Where the collaborative challenge comes in is how we allow others to influence our understanding of ourselves and how the world sees us. This connectedness with others and how they see us is important in the development of the rational and ethical self. As we established in Chapter 1, ethics takes place within the context of human relationships and therefore we need other people to reflect with us in order to develop our full potential as ethical nurses.

One of the key messages here is that reflection which takes place without a true knowledge of the situation and/or without the input of other people is likely to be flawed. That is without key reference points and perhaps a critical friend (someone who helps us question our assumptions) reflection may lead us to make decisions or form opinions which lack any real substance.

Complete Activity 2.2 to help you identify how you might use different orientations of reflection to help your development of ethical values and knowledge.

Activity 2.2 — *Reflection*

Read the following scenario and take a moment to think about what might be going on and then write a reflective entry using the dialectic (thinking about the political, social, ethical and use of power within the scenario) and the transpersonal (with regard to the development of self as an ethical practitioner) orientations.

There are some possible answers to all activities at the end of the chapter, unless otherwise indicated.

Case study: Raoul's concern with documentation in practice

Raoul is in the second year of his nurse training and is on placement in a busy surgical ward. He has just completed theoretical input about assessment and decision making in university and needs to find a patient to use as a case study for his assignment while on placement.

There are many theatre lists each day and the ward also has a number of orthopaedic patients because of a bed crisis. As these patients are recovering from anaesthesia, Raoul undertakes many nursing observations. He notices that patients who are over 24 hours postoperative seem to have similar trends in their observations. He assumes that this is a sign of their recovered status and thinks no more about it until he observes a first-year student nurse Lucy filling in the observation chart without having taken any readings or undertaken any observations. He challenges Lucy about this, whereupon she says this is what she observed healthcare assistants doing in her previous placement when patients were due to go home.

(continued)

continued . . .

> *Raoul uses the knowledge he gained on his assessment and decision-making module to discuss the implications of this behaviour with Lucy. He focuses on what the consequences might be for the patient and for Lucy and asks how this behaviour fits with ethical codes and her values.*
>
> *They explore together what might have prompted such behaviour. Time was viewed by both Raoul and Lucy as one factor. There was always too much to do. Lucy had worked a lot of her time with health-care assistants up until this point in her programme and she wanted to feel part of the team rather than 'rock the boat'. Raoul shared some of the information he had recently learned about ethical* **dilemmas***. He and Lucy reflected on how their values were developing as they progressed through their training. Lucy was appreciative that Raoul had shared his learning with her and thought about their discussion on her way home. She thought about what she would do differently. Raoul completed some reflective writing when he returned home that evening, exploring what he had learnt about his own progress from this episode.*

In reflecting on this scenario, you may have considered the knowledge bases that Lucy and Raoul were working from and their own sense of identity. You might also have explored what the ethical dilemmas were. What is clear in this scenario is the collaborative manner in which Raoul used his own previous reflections to help contribute to the development of Lucy's clinical and ethical understanding. At this point you are guided to another book in this series, *Reflective Practice in Nursing* (Howatson-Jones, 2016), whose final chapter considers critical reflection in the context of interrelationships between inner and outer worlds of learning.

Being able to reconcile your internal sense of self with external action is essential for your mental wellbeing and maintaining ethical actions in ways that are authentic. If you are inexperienced, it can be really helpful to do this with someone who is a qualified nurse (or a more experienced student, as in the case of Lucy) who can help to guide your reflection through critical questions. This can assist you to identify how situations are shaping your behaviour and how you might be influencing the behaviours expressed in the situation. These are reflexive responses which we move on to explore in more detail now.

One important way of interpreting this scenario, which sheds light on one of the key messages of this chapter, is that Lucy is working in a **deductive** manner; that is, she has seen a practice and wants to validate it because it is easy to do. She sees the patients' 'normal' observations as being a tool that allows them to go home but fails to consider that this might have very different consequences than those she has experienced to date – she works with what she 'knows'.

On the other hand, Raoul has considered the situation from first principles: he has been inductive. Raoul has taken his learning about the observations and applied it to this scenario; he has learnt through being educated and reflection that essentially making up results is not the right thing to do.

Concept summary: deductive and inductive reasoning

Deductive reasoning	Inductive reasoning
Top-down approach	Works from the bottom up
Begins with a theory of how things might be	Observes what is happening
Uses deduction to validate or discard the ideas	Uses abstract reasoning processes to consider different possibilities
Works with facts	Transferable to different situations

Reflexive responses in ethical decision making

Reflexive responses relate to being aware of how our actions impact on others. This requires being self-aware and knowing yourself, not in a **narcissistic** sense, but in knowing your values and beliefs and how these are brought to bear on situations, or develop through them (Titchen and McMahon, 2013). Johns (2006) describes this as *being mindful*, which means a concentrated self-awareness that encompasses thinking, feeling, being in the body and the world all at once. So when considering the right thing to do in a particular situation you need to think about:

- What do the people involved want?
- Are there conflicts between what is wanted?
- What meaning am I making of the problem and what is this based on?
- What are the political, social and regulatory influences on the situation?
- How does this feel?
- What resources do I have to offer?
- What are the potential outcomes of the various courses of action?
- What learning can I take from this?

Consider the following case study and then answer the questions at the end.

Case study: Ian's learning from critiquing research

Ian was in the second year of his nurse training. One of the assignments he needed to complete was a critique of a research article. He had been told about different critiquing frameworks and most of these considered ethics as one of the areas for critiquing research. Ian chose to critique a research article on medicines management practice.

(continued)

continued . . .

He read the article three times. The first time was a skim read to ascertain the main points; the second time was to check the main points against the critiquing framework; the third time was an in-depth read to develop critical discussion points. During his second read Ian noticed that the research had been passed by an ethics committee in its design phase which means that gaining access, informing partici-pants and establishing **consent** *were all addressed properly in the research design. However, during the in-depth read Ian discovered that one of the participants had disclosed making a drug error recently, when being interviewed by the researcher. The researcher was a nurse herself and was therefore regulated by the professional code of conduct. Ian was interested to note that instead of terminating the interview at that point, the interviewer had continued it by using guided reflection techniques. This had enabled her to determine that the patient had been managed appropriately as well as working with the partici-pant in an ethical way, demonstrating respect and supporting learning.*

Ian was intrigued by this as it seemed a deviation from the original research design plan. He reflected on why the researcher might have responded in this way. Ian considered that had the researcher termi-nated the interview it might have been perceived as judgemental. Instead it appeared that she had been allowing the participant to develop a reflexive narrative of events which was fuller and more detailed as a positive response. Ian thought about the ethics of this and decided to discuss this in his assignment.

Activity 2.3 — *Critical thinking*

Considering what you have already learned about ethics in the last chapter, what might have been the arguments Ian could have discussed in his assignment? What learning might Ian have taken from his discussion of this?

You might have considered the response of the researcher as being person-centred in caring for the participant in a respectful manner. At this point you are guided to another book in the series, *Patient Assessment and Care Planning in Nursing* (Howatson-Jones, 2015), and Chapter 7, which explores ethical dilemmas in practice. Being reflexive means remaining alert to cues, being able to work with difference and uncertainty and knowing yourself. Complete Activity 2.4 to set these ideas into the context of your life and practice.

Activity 2.4 — *Reflection*

Think about situations where you have had to respond to ethical uncertainty. How did it make you feel and why? What did you do? What did your decision mean for the other people involved? What were the outcomes? What did it tell you about yourself?

As this is based on your experience there is only a brief outline answer at the end of the chapter.

Being reflexive, therefore, is about building self-knowledge, seeing things from a number of different points of view, being clear about ethical issues and creatively exploring the options available to you and – this is important – to others. Being reflexive in this way mirrors the argument we make about the need for us to develop our ethical thinking in an inductive way; it is part of the art of nursing. Such artistry is part of the professional craft of nursing which is constantly being honed and adjusted to develop new ideas and practices (Finlay, 2008). Ethical problems always involve others in some way. Therefore, understanding our interactions is important to developing critical reflection on how we problem solve. The chapter now moves forward to consider this aspect in relation to ethical problem solving.

Collaborating in critically reflective ethical problem solving

Finlay (2008) suggests that collaboration is a *participatory dialogue* between practitioners which occurs when they are trying to solve problems. Such dialogues also need to include the patient who is perhaps the most important participant. This three-way dialogue is therefore a shared, person-centred, process of problem solving.

In order for such dialogues to be considered critical, they must be undertaken in a systematic manner which allows the problem to be explored and analysed from multiple different points of view. This multiplicity of views allows the participants to generate new perspectives which might inform what actions can be taken to influence the outcomes sought in the problem-solving process.

As such, critical questioning includes reviewing how personal morals and ethics might be influencing what is the best course of action to take in the situation being considered. This can feel challenging, especially when views which an individual really believes and takes for granted are held up for scrutiny and interrogated. Nevertheless, it is through these processes transformation is enabled and different ideas are possible. Consider the following activity and then answer the questions at the end.

Activity 2.5   *Critical thinking*

Cassie is in the second year of her nurse training and has a placement on a medical ward. An acquaintance – Jeremy – is admitted for stabilisation and review of his medication following an asthma attack. Cassie is aware that Jeremy occasionally smokes cannabis and that his present respiratory relapse may be due to this. She is worried about revealing this because the other staff might think that she also smokes cannabis, or that she might be breaking Jeremy's **confidentiality** by saying that he does smoke cannabis recreationally.

What should she do? Who should she involve? What might be the potential outcomes?

You might have considered that Cassie had real professional concerns about how she was viewed as a novice nurse. You might also have thought about what the main issue was here. In order to be systematic, critically reflective ethical problem solving involves:

- defining the problem – being clear about the problem and its parameters;
- identifying who is affected by the problem – the people involved;
- identifying how they are affected – what effects the problem is triggering, e.g. feelings;
- analysing different perspectives and options – looking at the alternatives available;
- developing an action plan – linking the options within a plan of how to proceed;
- implementing planned action in collaboration with others – putting the plan into practice;
- evaluating outcomes – reviewing the outcomes and changes to be made.

Such problem solving uses a mind-set that respects others as equals and listens to their point of view in an open way (Timmins, 2006). What this means is not assuming that we have the answers, or all the knowledge, but that there might be other ways of viewing the situation and of seeing the person or the problem. Working in collaboration with other professions requires open communication and understanding of different perspectives in order to come to a consensus that delivers a good outcome. Consider the next activity and answer the question at the end.

Activity 2.6   *Critical reflection*

David attended the radiology department for a therapeutic intervention dealing with a narrowing in an artery in his leg. David was a heavy smoker and had had a cigarette before coming into the treatment room. The therapeutic intervention involved placing a corrugated metal cylinder in the artery to keep it open and blood flowing through it. This was undertaken under X-ray control to ensure correct placement of the cylinder. The radiologist could smell the smoke on David and during the procedure began to tell him what would happen if he continued smoking and how expensive this procedure was in terms of equipment and staff. He suggested that David should get help from his general practitioner (GP) to stop smoking.

What do you think are the ethical issues in this scenario? Define the problem; identify those affected and how they are affected; analyse the different perspectives and options; develop an action plan of how to proceed.

The scenario highlights the importance of considering **positional power** when aiming to collaborate with others in ethical decision making. Good outcomes extend from open and transparent communication and self-knowledge. In essence, while the clinical message may be objective and clear, the specialist might have done well to reflect on the ethical message and the timing of the message before lecturing David when he was in a position of vulnerability.

Health and social care professionals often base such choices on rational thinking which looks for the best evidence of potential consequences. One of the key features of the scenarios presented is that the actors within them have chosen to consider their responses to the scenarios using the various reflective tools at their disposal. Muir (2004) asserts that this is a complex mental choice which is part of problem solving using normative thinking, which matches reasoning with action.

Increased conscious and conscientious application of decision making which pays heed to the physical and psychological context helps point the actors to a more considered route of action. The use of inductive, rather than more deductive, approaches to ethical decision making means that the outcomes of the activities, portrayed here, work to the benefit of all concerned. For example, the outcomes for Lucy and her learning are that she can see the potential risks to the patient of what she was doing as well as feel the loss of her professional integrity from her discussion with Raoul. This may guard against future concerns with 'fitting in' and ensure that she acts safely, effectively and, indeed, ethically.

The response of the researcher to the participant in Ian's scenario is more humane than simply following the rules in that there is an inductive response to the situation that supports longer-term learning. By demonstrating that the researcher valued the participant and showing how the situation could be explored and resolved in other ways, the researcher has helped Ian to learn alternative options for managing problems. This is important for his subsequent patient care and future career where different problems will present themselves.

Of course one of the benefits of approaching ethics in this reflective inductive manner is that the individual nurse or nursing student develops a more logical approach to problem solving. This considered approach will not only help in the sensible delivery of care, but also nurtures relationships, helps to grow the individual and allows the practitioner to start to make sense of the world of practice which can at times seem scary, illogical and inhumane.

In contrast, the issue with deductive approaches to ethical problem solving is that an action is taken and then the justification for the action is sought after the event. This leads to potentially negative consequences for the actors within the scenario. Individuals who make a snap decision may realise when trying to defend their action that it is indefensible; or that they are unhappy with their own explanation. Other people affected by the action may also feel aggrieved by what has occurred and fail to understand the underlying motives.

The scenarios in this chapter lay out how deductive ethical decision making is potentially risky for all concerned. Of course there is a need to be realistic, especially when operating in an acute or emergency situation, as delayed decision making might have deleterious consequences for all concerned.

Nevertheless, a lack of inductive reasoning in ethical decision making also suggests a lack of respect for people; it is not person-centred. If each person is an individual, then the things which motivate them and make them who they are unique and therefore each scenario and each individual deserves individual consideration and solutions. Reflecting in the moment takes account of individual considerations within a given situation and thus works with individuals' perspectives, while looking back at the actions taken allows working with all types of knowledge to come to a conclusion.

Another benefit of inductive ethical decision making is that it equips the individual nurse with the ability to respond ethically and congruently to novel situations and ethical dilemmas. This is because inductive reasoning works from foundational rules which are the same in any and every scenario; this is especially helpful in nursing where no two scenarios are the same and when healthcare provision is evolving and changing over time.

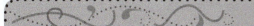

Chapter summary

This chapter has explored how personal values develop through the use of reflection in and on action and become embedded in different ways to support ethical problem solving and decision making. Through the scenarios and activities you have been encouraged to examine your own values and beliefs and to review how these are developing and becoming embedded. By continuing to explore your reflexive responses in different situations you will be able to develop knowledge of your own ethical decision making and what it is based upon. This is the inductive approach in action.

We have established that, in ethically challenging situations, inductive reasoning based on ethical principles and informed by reflection and reflexivity provides nurses with a coherent way of working out what is the ethical thing to do and how the decision they make will impact all of the players within the given scenario.

Activities: brief outline answers

Activity 2.2 Reflection

Raoul's reaction appeared to be based on his own values and beliefs of integrity and maintaining good practice. Lucy's seemed to be based more on a social model of doing the accepted thing to fit in. You might have written something about how macro politics from government-set targets can result in meaningless information being provided just to make sure the target is met. Equally, local politics in the way people interact with each other can result in power games where some people feel unable to challenge poor practice. The ethical dilemma which presents here is what is the best outcome and for whom? It is important to reflect on the surrounding events of the context and how to reconcile these factors in ways that are authentic. The learning which can come from such reflection and the development of a congruent safe and ethical practitioner are likely outcomes of reflecting on this scenario using a transpersonal perspective.

Activity 2.3 Critical thinking

Ian is likely to have discussed the researcher's response in relation to what professional code ethics require as well as with regard to caring for the participant. In particular, he is likely to focus on the fact that ethical decision making is a dynamic process requiring reflexive responses in order to meet competing demands and seek good outcomes. His arguments are likely to consist of the difference between rigidly following an ethical code and reflexively responding to situations by which new ethical insights might emerge. This is called inductive ethics because the ethics emerge from working and reflecting ethically in practice, whatever that practice may be.

Ian is likely to have learned that deviating from a set format does not mean that people are not behaving ethically; rather it suggests a reflexive response to the situation which is dynamic and in keeping with the moment. This can appear risky to those with less experience.

Activity 2.4 Reflection

You might have thought about sitting in on a friend's or relative's consultation, or times when you have not had sufficient resources to meet patients' needs, or when diagnostic information has been withheld until all tests are complete. You might have felt helpless because you could not share information, maybe even angry that what is needed is not available (see the discussion about moral stress in Chapter 1). You might have tried to reassure the person involved. The outcome is likely to depend on how authentic and accurate your information sharing was and this will also influence how you felt about yourself.

Activity 2.5 Critical thinking

Cassie might talk to Jeremy first to check her assumptions, as his asthma relapse may be completely unrelated to her suspicion that he has been smoking cannabis. If he has been smoking cannabis then she could encourage Jeremy to divulge this himself to aid his treatment. Nevertheless, Cassie also needs to be clear about her **duty of care** to Jeremy and that she will need to collaborate with the healthcare team to ensure the right treatment is given. Cassie could talk to her mentor about her concerns regarding the situation. The potential outcomes might be that Jeremy takes responsibility for his own narrative to ensure health professionals have accurate information on which to base his treatment options. The outcome of talking to her mentor might be that Cassie has an opportunity to explore her own taken-for-granted assumptions about the reason for Jeremy's admission and a clearer idea about how her own prejudices against smoking in general are influencing her assumptions about Jeremy's admission to hospital. Examining this with her mentor can help explore her ethical and moral thinking. Involving others in trying to problem solve is likely to reduce Cassie's anxiety, clarify the problem and deal with it effectively through wider experience.

Activity 2.6 Critical reflection

The problem is David's smoking, which is causing narrowing of his arteries requiring therapeutic intervention. David is affected by his smoking in terms of his arteries becoming narrowed. The radiologist is affected in that he has to treat David, but feels that this a problem of David's own making. The GP will be affected in offering David advice and resources to quit smoking. The public at large are affected in having to fund the treatment. The radiologist feels annoyed that resources are being used for someone who is able to avoid the problem developing. David does not feel equal to arguing with the radiologist as he is in a vulnerable position and unable to get away at this moment in time.

It appears that the radiologist is taking a controlling stance by telling David what he should do. His collaboration with David or the GP is not apparent. He has not considered David's perspective and possible reasons why he might be smoking. The alternatives available might be to find these out first before trying to proceed. The plan at present seems likely to fail as David might well be disinclined to listen. It may not be ethical to force opinions onto another person, especially when that person is in a vulnerable position. David is likely to take the message away that the radiologist will not treat him again if he is still smoking!

Further reading

Howatson-Jones, L (2015) *Patient Assessment and Care Planning in Nursing*, 2nd edn. London: Sage.
A holistic look at patient assessment.

Howatson-Jones, L (2016) *Reflective Practice in Nursing*, 3rd edn. London: Sage.
This book, which is aimed at the novice and more experienced practitioner, looks at different ways of developing analytical skills through personal and professional modes of reflection.

Jasper, M (2003) *Beginning Reflective Practice* (with Coursemate and ebook) (Nursing and Health Care Practice). London: Cengage learning Inc.
A well-tried and tested introduction to reflection.

Standing, M (ed.) (2010) *Clinical Judgement and Decision-Making in Nursing and Inter-Professional Healthcare.* Milton Keynes: Open University.

A more advanced, but accessible, look at decision-making models and theory.

Useful websites

www.businessballs.com/johariwindowmodel.htm

A quirky but very useful website for leadership theory; this page is about the Johari window referred to in this chapter.

Chapter 3
What ethics is and what ethics is not

Peter Ellis

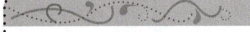

NMC Standards for Pre-registration Nursing Education

This chapter will address the following competencies:

Domain 1: Professional values

7. All nurses must be responsible and accountable for keeping their knowledge and skills up to date through continuing professional development. They must aim to improve their performance and enhance the safety and quality of care through evaluation, supervision and appraisal.

Domain 4: Leadership, management and team working

4. All nurses must be self-aware and recognise how their own values, principles and assumptions may affect their practice. They must maintain their own personal and professional development, learning from experience, through supervision, feedback, reflection and evaluation.

NMC Essential Skills Clusters

This chapter will address the following ESCs:

Care, compassion and communication

1. As partners in the care process, people can trust a newly registered graduate nurse to provide collaborative care based on the highest standards, knowledge and competence.

By entry to the register:

8. Demonstrates clinical confidence through sound knowledge, skills and understanding relevant to field.

Chapter aims

After reading this chapter you will be able to:

- discuss what factors influence your personal and professional ethics;
- describe what issues ought not to influence ethical decision making;
- explain how you derive your own personal ethical viewpoint;
- explore the interactions between various influences on your ethical activity.

In Chapter 1, we established something of the nature of ethics as it applies to our concept of ourselves, especially as nurses. This exploration led us to consider some issues around what our values are and how they are formed. We further explored how these might impact on our decision to become, socialise into, and remain nurses. In Chapter 2 we discussed how ethics should guide our decision making rather than be used a means of justifying decisions we have already made; that is, we suggested a model for inductive ethical decision making which put the use of ethical tools and reflection at the start and the heart of the ethical decision-making process.

In this chapter we will add to this understanding of ethics by exploring some of the influences which dictate the nature and diversity of ethical thinking and behaviour. We will explore some of the issues which go toward creating and explaining ethics and its place, and influence, in our day-to-day lives as well as on the society in which we live. This will require you to engage in some far-reaching thinking about who you are and what you value (as we did in Chapter 1) as well as reflecting on the influences on who you are and what you think about morality. This challenge requires us to take a holistic view of ethics and ethical life, considering the value and the impact of everyday understandings, beliefs and rituals which have a bearing on the ways in which we see and understand our world.

This chapter seeks to add some context to the discussion of personal values which we had in Chapter 1. Understanding the influences which shape us and give rise to our value sets allows us to explore whether these influences, and our resultant values, should form the basis of our personal and professional ethics; and conversely, whether they should not.

We are, if you like, going to explore some of the lenses which both colour and add depth to the ways in which we see and understand human activity; or, to put it another way, to look at some of the other influences on the creation of our moral and ethical understanding. Think of it like this: in Chapter 1 we thought about what our values are and how these might be moulded by being nurses; in this chapter we are taking the step of looking at what might mould these values in perhaps a more general sense as well as considering the other influences which have an impact on the ways in which we make ethical decisions.

Understanding influences on ethics

Why might it be important for us to understand the influences on our ethical thinking and what constitutes ethics in general? This important question is not as odd as it might at first seem. When we understand the influences on the ways we think and the influences on ethical norms and values we can start to understand how we, as individuals and collectively as nurses and members of a wider society, formulate what we consider to be ethical understandings. What is more, when we look to the influences on our ethical thinking we start to understand how ethics should operate – how we should put ethics into practice – as well as developing an understanding of how we might approach, and answer, new ethical questions and dilemmas.

Failure on the part of nurses to understand the influences on their decision making in general, and their ethical decision making in particular, may lead them to make decisions which are ill-informed and lack the sort of credibility which we associate with twenty-first-century evidence-based nursing. Take, for example, nurses brought up in the Roman Catholic tradition: their faith will impact greatly on the negativity they might feel about abortion. This negativity may contrast vastly with the opinions and beliefs of individuals brought up at the same time in the same community, but who are not Catholic, and who are perhaps more liberal in their view of abortion. The interesting question here is not whether one of these points of view is right or wrong; the important question is how the different influences on how they see the world lead them to their opposite viewpoints. What is more, it is important to discover whether or not they allow this viewpoint to influence the way in which they work and how they treat patients – expressly in this example women who are planning, are undergoing, or who have had a planned abortion.

Activity 3.1   *Reflection*

What have you experienced to date that has made a big impression on you, and what has shaped what you consider to be right and wrong? It might be people, such as teachers, or it might be an event. It may be losing a loved one or perhaps something you saw on the news like a natural disaster. What influences from your upbringing affect who you are today? For example your parents' beliefs, or indeed what they do for a living. Reflect on these influences, perhaps discuss them with a colleague or classmate, and look for similarities and differences in each other's ethical influences and beliefs.

Since the answers to this activity are personal to you, there is no specimen answer at the end of the chapter.

It is apparent there are many influences on the things we believe. Many of these influences come from our childhood when we listened to and took on board the beliefs and *knowledge* of our parents, teachers and friends. We perhaps failed to notice, and perhaps later acknowledge, these influences and, rather than moderate the impact they have on what we believe and who we become, we allow them to exert what may be undue influence on us.

Rationally as professionals, and aspiring professionals, the things we should allow to influence us as nurses are things which on reflection make sense. Or to put it another way, we should not allow ideas, understandings and other things to influence us until such time as we have had the opportunity to think about them and what they mean. In another book in this series, Ellis (2013, p. 18) argues that *informed nursing action [is] delivered with an understanding and appreciation of the complexity not only of the information associated with the medical management of a patient but also the complex nature of human interaction, beliefs and ethics.* This complexity exists not only in relation to evidence-based nursing practice – as is being described in the quotation – but in all aspects of nursing care delivery, whether it is driven by *evidence* or not.

The argument is at its core quite a simple one: once we understand the things which influence what we believe, what we know, what we feel and how we behave, we can start to take some control of them. Conversely, if we fail to understand the influences on our thoughts and behaviours, they control us. This corresponds well with the argument in Chapter 2 about using inductive reasoning to inform what we do ethically rather than acting first and seeking to justify our actions later.

In Chapter 1 we alluded to the idea of moral relevancy (that is, decisions which have a moral dimension) as opposed to decisions which should have no moral relevance. The argument made there was that some things are morally and ethically important and some things are not. So, for instance, how Rob behaves and how he speaks to people is morally relevant; where Rob comes from and his accent are not.

The argument being advanced here is that we not only need to identify what are morally relevant scenarios and behaviours, but also to identify the influences (both internal and external to ourselves) which control our thinking and responses to these. Subsequently we need also to decide which influences we should (morally) allow and which we should not.

Why understanding influencing factors is important

In the preceding section we highlighted the need to understand and be in control of influencers of ethical decision making. In this section and most of the rest of the chapter we will look in detail at some of the elements of day-to-day life which impact on the way in which we might make ethical decisions. At no stage is this exploration meant to be demeaning or to denigrate any beliefs or understandings we may hold as individuals; the **intention** is to prompt us as nurses to explore the influences on our ethical lives so that we might understand better not only ourselves, but also those about us.

As humans we experience similar situations, behaviours and emotional responses and therefore we are likely to develop similar views about the *rightness* or *wrongness* of some situations. Some of these shared views (perhaps about really heinous crimes like murder and genocide) are strongly bound and the linkages which bind us together as humanity are tight and not easily broken. Other views we hold may overlap with the views of others, but the extent to which this meeting of views occurs might vary (for example, what we feel constitutes reasonable force in self-defence) and this variance might change according to our personal experiences (being the subject of a violent crime) and perhaps news items (for example, the Tony Martin self-defence case – see Useful Websites, below).

Then there is the third area, an area in which some of us, although sharing some strong common views on other issues, will never see eye to eye. Ethical areas of strong disagreement might include abortion and **euthanasia** (see Chapter 7); debates around these subjects are often influenced by more individual opinions, beliefs and attitudes (Cox et al., 2013).

Activity 3.2 — *Reflection*

Think about how your opinion regarding something may have changed over time, for example how you might see being drunk after working in the emergency department or how you feel about euthanasia having had a work placement in a hospice. Has your view changed from what might be considered as being a commonly held view to one which is less common? Or perhaps it has changed from a view which you did not hold strongly to one which you now regard as being very important to you.

Since the answers to this activity are personal to you, there is no specimen answer at the end of the chapter.

The purpose of reflecting on the influences on the formation of our own ethical views and the ethical views of others is that it allows us to ask questions about what influences we should allow and what influences we should not.

For example, simple prejudice against gender, race or age does not provide a morally relevant reason to think negatively about people who seek cosmetic surgery on the NHS, whereas issues of vanity (as opposed to disturbed body image) might. Similarly, it may seem reasonable and moral to use public funds for treating injuries sustained while playing sport, but not necessarily for treating injuries sustained while carrying out a burglary.

Comparing one's own views with those of another allows us to test the credibility of the view we hold. Being prepared to challenge our own views and opinions is key to achieving a truly ethically active view on nursing – that is, an informed and inductive view.

Factors which influence ethical decision making

So far in this chapter we have identified that there are influences on ethical decision making and that it is important we are aware of what these are. In this section we will start to examine what some of these influences might be and how they might exert influence over the ways in which we make personal and professional ethical decisions.

What is apparent is that it is right some of the influences should have an impact on our ethical decision making while others should not; ethical decision making is not undertaken in a vacuum. As we saw before some things are morally relevant and some things are not, what is important is that we recognise this and act accordingly. Some of the key influences on both ethical theory and ethical decision making include:

- the law;
- societal norms;
- social etiquette;
- professional codes;
- religious beliefs;
- visual and aesthetic senses;
- experience;
- practicality.

All of these factors can and do play a part in the creation of our ethical selves and how we see the world and make ethical decisions. The exact influence of each of these factors will vary between people and situations.

Despite identifying the influences on ethical decision making as including all of the above, it is also important to explore what ethics is not or, perhaps more correctly, the extent of the influence which various factors should have on our ethical decision making. Some examples of common influences which perhaps should not be allowed to solely guide our ethical decision making include:

- religious ideologies;
- sentimentality;
- professional codes of conduct or ethics.

Allied to the fact that some factors should not be allowed to exert sole influence on our ethical development and decision making are some other important notions about what ethics is not including:

- being just for discussion;
- purely subjective;
- always relative.

Case study: personal ethics influencing practice

In 2012 the general practitioner Dr Richard Scott was called before a disciplinary panel of the General Medical Council after a patient complained that he was told to pray rather than receiving standard medical treatment for his mental health condition. Dr Scott's Christian ethics lead him to believe that prayer will help heal the sick. The ethical question remains, should he offer prayer instead of standard medical treatment to an individual who does not share his beliefs or in situations where prayer has not been shown to be of any medical benefit?

The rest of this chapter will look at each of the individual ideas identified in the list above. Where a general idea appears in both lists (e.g. in relation to ideas such as religion and codes of conduct) the idea will be merged under one heading to allow some clarity in the argument being created. You should consider each idea and use them to inform your emerging picture of what ethics is and what it is not.

The law

On initial inspection it may seem that the law and ethics are virtually the same thing. Law is about protecting people in society and about attaining **justice** for the many in much the same way in which we identified why ethics are important in Chapter 1. But there are subtle and important differences; once you as a nurse start to understand these differences, the importance of ethics in guiding your day-to-day practice will become even more apparent.

The first difference between law and ethics is a simple one: law exists in a written form as set guidelines for behaviour; ethics does not, at least not to the same degree as law. What is of note, however, is that there is not a law for everything, but – and this is an important but – there is an ethical response to *all* situations and activities which involve human activity.

In much of the UK (Scotland being slightly different) **common law** operates. Common law uses a system whereby actions are judged in a court of law in comparison to previous similar cases which set a **precedent** for the decision the judge will make. Some law in the UK is subject to **statute**; that is, law which is decided upon in Parliament.

What common and statute law share in common is that they tend to be responsive to events which have already happened. It is not possible to pass a law or create a precedent for an action or activity which has yet to take place or for scenarios which have not been foreseen. In the healthcare setting then, laws to guide action would not be enough as they would not be able to keep pace with changing technology, advances in care, changing societal norms and the complexities of individualised patient care.

Ethical guidelines and codes of conduct, on the other hand, provide what Beauchamp and Childress (2012) call *scope*; that is, guidance within which nurses can operate. Ethical codes and guidelines do not operate as definitive rules, as might the law; rather they present general rules within which nurses might act; if the law is a narrow path which nurses need to walk, then ethical codes are a multilane highway. On this broad highway it is correct to follow any of the lanes; the hard shoulder represents grey areas (dilemmas), while stepping off the highway onto the grassy verge is always wrong. In some respects this metaphor captures the idea that ethics is often, but not always, situational. On the other hand, the law very rarely is.

Activity 3.3   *Critical thinking*

In England, Scotland and Wales the upper gestational age for abortion is set at 24 weeks and has been since 1990, except in exceptional circumstances. In 1967, when the Abortion Act was first enacted, the upper gestational age for abortion was set at 28 weeks

(continued)

continued...

(Select Committee on Science and Technology, 2007). The change in legislation was a direct response to changes in the viability of the unborn child, which was in itself a direct response to changes in medical technology which made it possible to keep younger and younger neonates alive.

Given this observation, do you think that all legislation should be driven by medical advances such as this; or conversely do you think the law should place restrictions on medical advances?

There are some possible answers to all activities at the end of the chapter, unless otherwise indicated.

Activity 3.3 points us in a very controversial direction, whereby medical advances dictate law. In respect to the abortion debate the controversy is still very much alive as there is much debate about whether to admit newborns at 24 and 25 weeks into neonatal intensive care (Vavasseur et al., 2007) as they are at the limits of survivability. Such controversy makes for difficult law making as the law is now responsive and fails, unlike ethical codes, to provide some immediate guidance for practice.

Of course, in some situations there is no law, be that up-to-the-minute legislation or dated; but, and this is again an important but, *ethics* apply in every possible situation. This is no anomaly – laws are made to guide actions in a predetermined and set manner, but life does not proceed in a predetermined and set manner. Nowhere is this truer than at the point of care. Controversies arise and dilemmas present themselves on a daily basis; these dilemmas require action, often immediate, and therefore cannot be left for the law to decide.

Activity 3.4   *Reflection*

Consider a recent issue from practice which caused some ethical debate among the team. What were the issues involved? Who was affected? What were the ethical and moral issues involved? Were there any legal precedents which could inform what the team did? Was a consensus reached? How did this make you feel?

Since the answers to this activity are personal to you, there is no specimen answer at the end of the chapter.

Unusual circumstances in care arise out of changes in practice, new technology, patients' choices and perhaps where there are questions about an individual patient's **capacity** (see Chapter 6) to make a decision. Learning to reflect on these issues, asking questions like those posed in Activity 3.4, is an important part of growing your own ethical awareness and development of values to guide your nursing practice.

Of course, where there is law to inform practice, this should almost invariably take precedence over any other form of decision making.

Social etiquette/norms

Social norms seem like an odd example of issues which might inform ethical thinking in nursing. After all, social norms are constantly evolving and differ between communities and cultures and in time and place. If we accept the notion put forward in Chapter 1, that we live in social groups to better our existence and that ethical activity within these social groups helps to protect our quality of life, then it is apparent that society plays an important role in how ethical norms are derived.

In statistics, there is an idea called regression to the mean. This idea states that if you ask enough people to guess a quantity (for example, the number of sweets in a jar) you will eventually reach a state where the mean (average) of all of their answers is in fact the true number and this will continue to hold true thereafter. What this illustrates is the moderating influence of a group of people. In the case of the development of social norms and etiquette, the moderating influences of large groups of people (with various beliefs, attitudes and opinions) will usually mean that the right behaviour (social etiquette) and the right understanding (social norm) will be arrived at over a period of time as a result of the influence of the input of the various members of society.

Of course this is a little over-simplified but the ideas are on the whole true. Consider the occasions when you have chosen not to drop litter or make an illegal manoeuvre in your car, not because you did not want to (because they are often easier than the alternative) but because someone else was watching. We are all influenced to a greater or lesser extent by the fact that other people are watching what we do.

Activity 3.5 *Reflection*

Consider your last positive interaction with someone who was providing a service, such as in a restaurant or bar. Why was it positive and what did it make you feel about the person and the service s/he was providing? Now consider the last time someone in a service role upset you. What did the person do or say to upset you? How did this make you feel about the service? If you cannot think of an example of your own, revisit the case study featuring Manu in Chapter 2.

What appears to be going on with etiquette and ethics is some interplay between behaving politely (i.e. following etiquette) and the ethicality of the individual – perhaps because both politeness and ethicality reflect respect for other persons and their **autonomy**. Of course this is a crude barometer, but nevertheless it is probably true that ethical individuals also exercise good manners in their interactions with others.

Professional codes

In the first part of this chapter we suggested that ethics is informed by, but not the practice of quoting, professional codes of conduct. One of the truisms about any code of conduct is that it is, in reality, at best only a general guide to behaviour. Take for example *The Code: Professional Standards of Practice and Behaviour for Nurses and Midwives*, published by the Nursing and Midwifery Council in 2015, which exhorts us to prioritise people and '*make their care and safety your main concern and make sure that their dignity is preserved and their needs are recognised, assessed and responded to*' (p. 4). On first glance this is simple to follow. But look again: what does *prioritise people* mean and how do we ensure *their dignity is preserved?*

If we were to follow set rules, as might be laid down in law, then prioritising people and preserving dignity would mean following a prescribed action or set of actions. There would be little room for manoeuvre and, anyway, can this really mean we do the same thing in every situation?

As with the law, a code cannot pre-empt every eventuality; what it can do is provide a general basis for action and ways of behaving. For example, we know that respecting someone's dignity means providing them with privacy and maintaining confidentiality, but in an emergency situation this can be scaled down as we respond to their very real immediate needs. As with the law, where the ideas contained with the code are clear and the situations well defined, then codes of conduct provide perhaps the most important driver for decision making. Sometimes codes of conduct provide good reasons for the ways in which we might choose to act as nurses and at other times they provide a convenient excuse!

What is clear is that as nursing students the code of conduct is a good guide to the general levels of behaviour you should adopt, but they are not a replacement for the development of ethical awareness.

Religion

For many people of faith, their religion is the first port of call for an answer to a moral or ethical question. While this may be right and proper for us in our day-to-day lives, within the scope of our practice as nurses this may prove to be controversial at best (see the earlier case study about Dr Richard Scott). On other occasions religious teachings and prescribed behaviours have had a profound influence on more secular (worldly) approaches to ethics, morality and social norms because of the way they have become embedded in national and international culture.

One of the key differences between ethical acts which are professional and personal in nature and those which are influenced by a religious intent is the motivation which underlies them (Alkire, 2007). For people of faith following the instructions of their faith, and indeed the actions of their prophets and deities, can in itself prove to be enough of a motivation to act in what might be described as a religious duty-bound (but nevertheless ethical) manner.

For people of no faith, the motivation to act ethically may come from some other influence such as their upbringing, their personality or from a worldlier set of ethical motivators. Such motivation could also be duty-based, like that of the religious individual, but as we have seen in Chapter 1 and as we shall see elsewhere in this book, there are multiple approaches to ethical thinking and behaviours.

While religious belief no doubt has a positive impact on the ethical life of individual nurses and nursing in general, and, in the West, we are certainly affected by both Judaism and Christianity (for example, the ten commandments and common statements like 'do unto others as you would have them do to you'), there remain some issues with relying too much on religion in the professional setting.

The first issue is being able to justify the imposition of our own religious views on other people who either have no religious belief or are of a different faith. This may lead to tensions with respecting individual autonomy and the nursing philosophy of person-centred care. This religious bias may manifest in the ways in which we make decisions which may or may not be in the patient's best interests, but which rather represent the healthcare professional's own religious point of view. For example, a nurse who is a Roman Catholic and whose conduct is purely motivated by her faith may feel she cannot educate a young woman about the use of contraception because her religion forbids it.

Second, as healthcare professionals, we may not agree with the religious convictions of others and may regard the decisions they make as inferior to those we might make. The classic example is that of the Jehovah's Witness who refuses a blood transfusion even though it will in all probability lead to that person's death.

Concept summary: the Jehovah's Witness view on blood transfusions

Jehovah's Witnesses believe that the Old Testament of the Bible as well as God's position as the 'giver of life' forbids them from having blood transfusions and blood products, even in the most extreme circumstances. Clearly there will be occasions when a Jehovah's Witness attends hospital in an emergency situation when it would be in that person's medical best interests to have a blood transfusion or some other blood product (**www.jw.org**).

Clearly the place of faith and religion in the working life of the nurse is a controversial area. One of the difficulties for student nurses who come to nursing with established belief systems is learning to strike the balance between what they believe and how they are allowed to act in the workplace.

Aesthetic senses and sentimentality

As nurses we are socialised from the early stages in our career to be empathetic and sympathetic. These qualities are essential if we are to have meaningful relationships with our patients. It is very easy, however, for empathy and sympathy to become sentimentality. Being sentimental and relying on our **aesthetic** senses is, on the one hand, a positive trait but, on the other, it may cloud our judgement and cause us to approach potentially ethical questions in the wrong way.

In Chapter 2, we discussed the need to approach ethical decision making in an inductive manner; that is, to allow the principles to guide our decisions rather than using principles to try to underpin decisions we have already made. One of the key dangers of sentimentality and aesthetic approaches to ethics is that they tempt us to make our ethical decisions based on what we feel and what looks good rather than based on what we know or have at the very least considered.

There is, however, an important point to be considered here, illustrated in Activity 3.6.

Activity 3.6 — *Critical thinking*

Consider the following scenario.

Julie is a student nurse on placement in a nursing care home. Part of the home provides care for people with dementia. Julie has no experience of dementia care and is quite anxious about working in the dementia unit and has no idea what to expect. On her first day Julie is tasked to work with a care assistant, Justine. The shift progresses well and Julie starts to feel comfortable in her new surroundings. At tea time one of the male patients, Gerald, becomes aggressive and refuses his food and lashes out at the staff trying to feed him. Justine responds by taking hold of one of his arms and restraining him while another care assistant, Ben, takes hold of the other. Justine tells Julie to feed Gerald while they are restraining him. Julie is reluctant. Justine tells Julie: 'This is what we do or he will starve'. Gerald is clearly distressed. Julie is not sure about whether she should feed Gerald against his will, but is anxious he should not starve. What should she do?

What this activity indicates is that, on some occasions at least, the aesthetic and sentimental senses we have can provide us with answers as to how we might act even when this activity appears to fly in the face of the rational argument. Consider the nature of the argument put forward by the emotivists in the following concept summary.

Concept summary: Aesthetics and emotivism

Aesthetic responses to ethical situations belong to a school of ethical thought sometimes called **emotivism**. Emotivists claim that our values are firmly rooted in our emotional responses to situations and therefore ethical judgement is little more than an expression

(continued)

(continued)

of an opinion of like or dislike, approval or disapproval. One form of emotivism is rooted in **positivism**. Positivism states that we can only truly know those things which we can detect and test through our senses. Since we cannot sense ethical choices and they are not testable using our senses, they are not therefore truly knowable. Ethical choices and opinions are therefore no more than mere attitude or opinion.

Of course there are really big problems with basing what we do and how we justify it purely on our emotional response to situations. In healthcare much of what we do involves working with people who are in pain or distressed and some of what we do to help them might cause further pain or distress. Take, for example, the pain and distress caused to a baby who is being vaccinated. On face value there is little difference between this and the force feeding of Gerald. Both activities are done with the express aim of doing something positive for the patient; the only difference is no one would claim the act of vaccinating the baby had any negative moral dimensions even though it caused pain and distress.

Julie's reluctance to get involved with force feeding is a good example of how emotivism can provide us with a good moral guide. There is a clear lack of congruity between what Julie is being asked to do and her values (see Chapter 1) and what appears to her to be the right thing to do. In this scenario, the appearance of what is being done as being wrong is a good instinct as, despite claims to the contrary, force feeding another human being in this manner shows what can only be described as a lack of respect for that person.

All that said, the care assistants do not share Julie's revulsion at what they are doing, but this does not mean they are necessarily evil. The reframing of what we find acceptable and what appears to us to be the right and wrong thing to do can happen as a result of power being exerted over us or prolonged exposure to increasingly tenuous ethical practices – acculturation (see Chapter 1). The need to be alert to and nurture our value base in order to maintain our aesthetic ethical compass is therefore a major challenge facing nurses.

Experience

In Chapter 1, we defined ethics as *a practical art/science which helps to guide our activity in day-to-day life and, more specifically for us, nursing practice.* We have seen through some of the examples and activities within the book that ethics is part of the day-to-day experience of the nursing student and furthermore we have seen in some of the examples, especially within Chapter 2, that the guidance the student needed in order to do the right thing came from other people who had more nursing experience.

Clearly the accruing of experience as a nurse does not make us more ethical in itself. What experience does do is provide opportunities for us to reflect on, and in, action, identifying ways of working which are congruent with our values. That is to say, we can use our bank of experience to help guide how we might adapt what we do and how we might act in the future.

Of course the converse can also be true, especially when nurses allow themselves to become involved in poor care. Poor care starts to form the basis of their normal experience and they then become immune to it – see the following case study.

Case study: the Mid Staffordshire Inquiry

The Francis Report into the failings at Mid Staffordshire NHS Foundation Trust (Francis, 2013) makes some key observations about how poor care can come to be seen as the norm:

The negative aspects of culture in the system were identified as including:

- *a lack of openness to criticism;*
- *a lack of consideration for patients;*
- *defensiveness;*
- *looking inwards, not outwards;*
- *secrecy;*
- *misplaced assumptions about the judgements and actions of others;*
- *an acceptance of poor standards;*
- *a failure to put the patient first in everything that is done.*

In the example of Mid Staffordshire, the underlying poor culture had become so pervasive that it started to take precedence over what the staff there knew to be right. This demonstrates that, while experience is a good starting point for thinking about ethicality, it is not, on its own, enough.

Practicality/just for discussion

This may seem like an unlikely element of the ethical decision-making process but, as we have seen, ethics is a practical pursuit and there seems little point in making decisions which lack practical application. In his famous book *Practical Ethics*, Peter Singer (2011, p. 2) makes the important observation that: *an ethical judgement which is no good in practice must suffer from a theoretical defect … for the whole point of ethical judgements is to guide practice.*

What Singer is alluding to here, and the point this book makes time and time again, is that ethics is grounded in the real world and the decisions we take, especially as nurses, impact real people. Ethics does not occur in a vacuum and is therefore not just for discussion.

Subjective/relative

Subjectivity refers to how different people may view the same occurrence, such as an ethical dilemma, in different ways, while relativity refers to the ethicalness of a decision or action being based in the exact context of the situation. Clearly some elements of ethicality change over time and due to changes in society, medical advances, technological changes and new understandings. Examples of this might include the reduction in the gestational age at which abortion is acceptable due to knowledge which increased the viability of foetuses of much earlier gestation. Such changes do not make the ethics relative or subjective per se; what they do is serve to increase the importance of practicality in the ethical decision-making process. Whether abortion is right or wrong is not subjectively at question here, but the timeframe during which it might be ethical to undertake abortion is.

A further problem with accepting relativism or subjectivism as acceptable in ethical thought is that to do so would mean we could never address unethical behaviour. In Activity 3.6 we saw Julie thinking that it is wrong to force feed a patient with dementia, while Justine thinks exactly the opposite. Subjectivists might claim they are both right; but clearly this cannot be the case – although there are often ethical scenarios in which there is more than one right answer.

Case study: Dr Harold Shipman

Dr Harold Shipman was a general practitioner who worked in Hyde, Greater Manchester. In January 2000 he was found guilty of the murder of 15 of his patients, although it is suspected that he murdered up to 250. His usual mechanism of killing them was to use diamorphine injections. Many of Shipman's victims were terminally ill and, while Shipman provided no explanation for what he had done before he committed suicide in 2004, it is widely believed that he may have thought what he was doing was providing justifiable euthanasia to his victims.

The case of Shipman provides one clue as to why subjectivity in ethical thinking has to be viewed with considerable suspicion. While Shipman may have thought what he was doing was the right thing, there is no record of him having ever asked any of his victims whether they wanted to be euthanised. Subjectively he might lay claim to be 'doing the right thing' but this is clearly not the case.

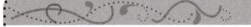

Chapter summary

In this chapter we have explored some of the influences on ethical decision making. We have seen that some influences exert a legitimate influence over the way in which decisions are made while others either do not or should not. It is because of the complexity of influences, especially within the clinical setting, that consideration of ethical issues in nursing requires some considerable effort.

The challenge for nursing students trying to construct an understanding of ethics for themselves is in seeing into, and sometimes past, the impact of previous experience, beliefs and understanding when engaging with the development of a truly ethical self.

Activities: brief outline answers

Activity 3.3 Critical thinking

Clearly it is not possible for the law to anticipate all advances in medical science as it is not possible for medical advances always to tailor themselves to ambiguous law. There are some issues which as a society we may decide we do not want medicine to explore (e.g. gender choice in in vitro fertilisation perhaps) because the moral repugnance of choosing gender (except perhaps where this is linked to some life-limiting disease) is something we as a society hold to be more important than science for science's sake.

In contrast, heavy-handed legislation which prevents advances in science may impact on survival and quality of life and so the interaction between law and science needs to be managed with a much lighter hand.

Activity 3.5 Reflection

Often when people providing a service upset us it is because of their manner. We consider them to be rude and therefore bad at what they do. When they are polite and helpful we consider them to be good. But is this true? Is our opinion at least in part coloured by the behaviour so that we overlook other aspects of the service, such as getting what we wanted or value for money. What appears clear is that the way we behave is at least as important as what we do and therefore the contribution of etiquette to our feelings of goodness or badness (ethicalness); or is it that people doing the right thing can be seen to be doing so?

Activity 3.6 Critical thinking

This is a difficult situation for two reasons: first, Julie does not know what is normal and, second, she knows that Gerald needs some nutritional input. Because of her lack of experience Julie has to rely on her aesthetic senses which tell her that force feeding a patient with dementia is wrong. The sentimental/ aesthetic view in this case acts as a conscience. This conscience tells Julie, quite rightly, that something about this does not look right. The rationalisation of the force feeding might appear to have some validity but at the end of the day Gerald is a human being and should be treated with humanity. Julie needs to discuss this situation as a matter of urgency with the home manager, and if she remains unsure it would be wise for her to escalate the issue to her personal tutor or link lecturer. If there is no satisfactory resolution to this issue this sort of event might constitute a reason for informing the local adult safeguarding team.

Further reading

Cranmer, P and Nhemachena, J (2013) *Ethics for Nurses: Theory and Practice.* Milton Keynes: Open University Press.
Chapter 1 gives a useful overview.

Singer, P (2011) *Practical Ethics*, 3rd edn. Cambridge: Cambridge University Press.
The first chapter especially sets out a fantastic overview of influences on ethical thinking.

Useful websites

jima.imana.org/article/viewFile/5245/38_3-3
This is an interesting paper on the influence of Judaism, Catholicism and Islam on medical ethics.

www.jw.org
Look here to understand better the Jehovah's Witness view of medical interventions.

news.bbc.co.uk/1/hi/3009769.stm
The Tony Martin case is examined: Tony Martin shot dead a teenager who was burgling his home. This article explores the thorny issue of self-defence in the home and what might and might not constitute reasonable force.

Chapter 4
Theories of ethics

Peter Ellis

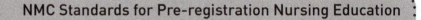

NMC Standards for Pre-registration Nursing Education

This chapter will address the following competencies:

Domain 1: Professional values

1. All nurses must practise with confidence according to *The Code: Professional Standards of Practice and Behaviour for Nurses and Midwives* (NMC, 2015), and within other recognised ethical and legal frameworks. They must be able to recognise and address ethical challenges relating to people's choices and decision making about their care, and act within the law to help them and their families and carers find acceptable solutions.

2. All nurses must practise in a holistic, non-judgemental, caring and sensitive manner that avoids assumptions, supports social inclusion; recognises and respects individual choice; and acknowledges diversity. Where necessary, they must challenge inequality, discrimination and exclusion from access to care.

Domain 4: Leadership, management and team working

6. All nurses must work independently as well as in teams. They must be able to take the lead in coordinating, delegating and supervising care safely, managing risk and remaining accountable for the care given.

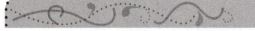

NMC Essential Skills Clusters

This chapter will address the following ESCs:

Care, compassion and communication

1. As partners in the care process, people can trust a newly registered graduate nurse to provide collaborative care based on the highest standards, knowledge and competence.

Organisational aspects of care

16. People can trust the newly registered graduate nurse to safely lead, coordinate and manage care.

> **Chapter aims**
>
> After reading this chapter you will be able to:
>
> * critically discuss the theories which inform ethical thinking;
> * consider how theory might inform your own practice;
> * identify the pros and cons of some ethical theories;
> * start to understand the nature of ethical decision making in nursing.

Introduction

Having a basic understanding of some of the key theories which inform ethical decision making is fundamental to being able to think about, discuss and use ethics in our nursing practice. One of the arguments contained in this book is that an understanding of ethics, and ethical theory, should precede any ethical decision making. That is to say, it is probably good sense and good practice to consider the theories of ethics which might apply to a situation before coming to a decision about what is right and what is wrong, what is ethical and what is not and therefore how to act in any given scenario. Knee-jerk reactions to new scenarios may prove to be wrong in time, so avoiding such reactions is perhaps wise.

In Chapter 2 inductive reflective thinking was explored in some detail. Adopting an inductive approach to ethical thinking allows us as professionals to put thought before action. Thinking first and acting later is an important element of evidence-based professional practice, as is argued in Chapter 3, and as such may help us in a manner which is not only professional but also ethically justifiable.

There are a very large number of ethical theories and ways of thinking in general which inform ethical decision making. Having an understanding of some of these theories, the basis behind them and the ways in which they are applied in practice, will help to inform nurses' day-to-day decision making.

This chapter will explore some of the key ethical theories and approaches prominent in western ethics. These explorations are not meant to be exhaustive nor are the discussions about each approach complete; there are two good reasons for this. The first is that this would take too long to do and the second is that this book is focused on applying ethics to practice, not exploring ethics as an academic topic.

Understanding approaches to ethics

In order to understand the various approaches to ethics, it is worth thinking about the nature of activity. All activity starts with a thought, a plan or, more properly, an intention. Even decisions which are made quickly in response to rapid stimuli are made to fulfil some form of intention. Intention may be something straightforward and easy to understand. Common human intentions include avoiding pain or self-preservation (as we saw in reference to Hobbes in Chapter 1). Intention may be a more psychological process, something which we deliberate on and spend time thinking about, such as the intention to develop, or preserve, the way in which people see you – for example, as a person with integrity. Even very simple actions, such as turning on a light, start with an intention; in this case the intention is not really just to turn on the light, but more properly it is about lighting up a room, a person or an object.

In this way we can see that intention precedes everything we do. Another way to think about it is to consider how we judge individuals in relation to what we consider to be their motives for doing something. Motives and intentions are the underlying reasons which cause us to behave in this way or that, undertake this action or that action. What should be clear here is that the intent underlying an act needs to be thought through before we make a judgement about what is happening (see the discussion about the **doctrine of double effect** in Chapter 7).

After intention comes the action. The action is whatever we choose to do, sometimes referred to as an **act of commission**. Very often in philosophical and ethical theory we refer also to inaction, things we choose not to do – also known as **acts of omission**. Either way these are provable as activity or inactivity and can be seen – witnessed – by others.

Concept summary: omission, commission and intent

Smith will inherit a lot of money if his 6-year-old cousin dies. One evening Smith sneaks into the bathroom and drowns his cousin who is taking a bath.

Jones also stands to inherit a lot of money if his 6-year-old cousin dies. One evening Jones sneaks into the bathroom and finds his young cousin drowning; he does nothing to save him.

Smith kills his cousin in an act of commission. Jones kills his cousin in an act of omission.

While the one act requires a wilful positive action and the other does not, the intent is the same. Most ethical thinkers agree there is little to choose between the two on an ethical basis.

(Adapted from Rachels, 1975)

Some actions, either of *commission* or *omission*, are just the right thing to do. For example, as a rule telling the truth is the proper way to behave. As an act, and regardless of consequences in this view, truth telling is good. So one view of ethics might be that we should always undertake actions which are *the right thing to do*.

Finally, for all intended and executed actions, or inactions, there are consequences. You might find this easier to think about in terms of cause and effect – for everything we do there is an outcome. So even a simple task, let's return to the turning on of the light, is simplistically a three-phase activity: the desire to switch on the light (the intention), the flicking of the switch (the action) and the actual lighting of the room (the consequence).

What bearing does this have on ethics and ethical thinking? Quite simply, if we are to consider how we might judge what people do, we need to consider activity in its entirety. The actions of people are not disconnected from the choices they make nor are they disconnected from the outcomes of the action. One thing we learn as children is that all actions have consequences, but some actions attract displeasure because of the act itself, such as lying or hitting, while other actions lead to displeasure in others because of their consequences, such as name calling which leads to a child crying, or failing to clear away toys which leads to someone tripping and being hurt. What separates these activities is, most often, intent. One justification we learn very early in life is to lay claim to the fact that 'I didn't mean that to happen!'

So where does this leave us? These ideas neatly frame three of the most commonly described and discussed theories of **normative ethics** – the study of ethical action – they are **consequentialism**, **non-consequentialism** and **virtue ethics**. Because of their central importance in understanding western ethics in particular, this chapter will examine these three schools of ethical thought, employing some examples to illustrate their use as well as examining some of the arguments made against them in the ethical literature.

Concept summary: normative ethics

The notion of normative ethics refers to attempts to discover the rightness or wrongness of an action by reference to the action itself. Normative ethics then seeks to establish some consistency to ethical questions posed within any given context. The types of questions normative ethics might ask are therefore:

- What is good and evil?
- What is right and wrong?
- How ought one to act ethically?

Because of the central importance of these ethical theories to the arguments made elsewhere in this book and in the wider ethics literature, students are encouraged to ensure they understand the nature of each of these ethical schools of thought before they proceed further with their reading.

Consequentialism

Consequentialism is a school of moral thought which ascribes the *rightness* of an action to be determined by the consequences of the action. What this means in action is that *the ends justify the means* or that it is not the action itself which is important, but the consequences of the action. For a consequentialist, then, a good, or moral, action is one which has a positive outcome. Some definitions of consequentialism also refer to inaction, not doing something, *an omission*, as a route to achieving a good outcome.

Consequentialism is popular in political thought because one of its central tenets is *achieving the greatest good for the greatest number.* Despite the appearance of being based on sound bites, consequentialism is a serious ethical philosophy. The predominant school of consequential thought is called **utilitarianism**. Considering consequentialism in terms of utilitarianism is helpful on many levels as utility (the word root of utilitarianism) means usefulness. Utilitarian ethics are therefore characterised by their *usefulness.*

This leaves us with an important question: what does useful mean and to whom should it be useful? This question points us to one of the key positives and one of the key negatives of this ethical theory. The definition of what is useful and to whom is a matter for considerable debate, while the notion that ethical actions have a positive benefit for a large group of individuals rather than an individual is a strong positive.

So where did this all come from? Jeremy Bentham, widely considered to be the founding father of utilitarianism, based his philosophy around a **moral calculus** (equation) which said that an action was good if it maximised pleasure and minimised pain. For Bentham (1781) the desire to avoid pain and maximise pleasure explained why people make the choices they do as well as providing a moral justification for the choices made. Bentham's brand of utilitarianism is known as **act utilitarianism** – the actions which people do are only right if they maximise pleasure in any given situation. So, for example, if on this occasion lying would bring about the greatest pleasure and minimise pain then on this occasion lying is the right act.

Activity 4.1   *Decision making*

Maureen is a 72-year-old woman admitted to your ward for investigations into weight loss. It is discovered that she has a late-stage terminal cancer and has only a few weeks to live. On finding out this news her husband tries to prevent the nursing and medical staff from telling her; he argues the news will only upset her and telling her nothing and allowing her to come home will make her happy. Using act utilitarianism as your guide, what might you do?

There are some possible answers to all activities at the end of the chapter, unless otherwise indicated.

Activity 4.1 points to the fact that, because outcomes are often uncertain, act utilitarianism, which takes into account only the action under examination, can often be less than helpful in making real-life decisions. In large part this is because this approach to using utilitarianism only takes into account the situation directly in front of us and it pays no heed to the experience and insight gained in previous similar situations. The other massive issue here is the fact that regardless of what her husband thinks, it just feels wrong to lie to an adult who is capable of making their own choices.

John Stuart Mill (1789) subsequently adapted the notion of utilitarianism to make the calculus more qualitative. Mill believed some pleasures, such as intellectual pursuits, were more important than others and therefore deserved a higher score when undertaking the moral calculus equation.

In Mill's view, utilitarian actions, and hence therefore the utilitarian equation, should not be confined to singular events, but to rules which if followed would benefit all people generally speaking. Mill's school of utilitarianism is called **rule utilitarianism** and it suggests that people should follow the rule which will lead to the greatest happiness.

Rule utilitarianism suggests the wellbeing of an individual is of prime importance. Happiness is only truly achieved by following rules which promote the happiness of everyone – remembering, however, that some things are more important when calculating this than others.

Activity 4.2   *Decision making*

Reread the scenario in Activity 4.1. Using rule utilitarianism as your guide, what might you say to Maureen's husband?

Rule-based utilitarianism captures something more than act utilitarianism in relation to this type of scenario as it seeks answers which have more meaning and which may apply beyond the individual scenario under consideration. This in some respects overcomes the situational unsustainability of act utilitarianism which does not consider the ongoing context in which similar decisions have to be made repeatedly. In this respect rule-based utilitarianism addresses the key concern about act utilitarianism in that it can at least recognise the ongoing impact of a course of action and what it might mean in a broader context.

Consequences are of great importance to us as nurses in that we seek to provide positive outcomes and to this end we assess needs and plan our care with specific outcomes in mind. Estefan (2011, p. 35) makes the observation:

> *Happiness and pleasure are physical and psychological phenomena amenable to nursing interventions; for example, implementing nursing measures to reduce pain and discomfort. Importantly, promoting happiness and pleasure for patients goes beyond physical interventions.*

Estefan goes on to challenge nurses to stop and take stock of who we are and how we interact with patients using the consequentialist approach.

Activity 4.3   *Reflection*

What do you think about the idea of increasing happiness and pleasure for patients? What are the boundaries in relation to this? What things have you done for patients, their family or other visitors recently which served to increase their happiness, but which might not, strictly, have been nursing actions?

Since the answers to this activity are personal to you, there is no specimen answer at the end of the chapter.

The answer to Activity 4.3 in part lies within the context of the fact that we, as care professionals, get to understand what the likely consequences are of some of the interventions we undertake. In this context, planning activity towards a known goal is a somewhat simpler task than ethical decision making using consequentialism. There are also some simple actions we undertake which add to the pleasure, or if you like the experience, of patients and their visitors. Simple acts of kindness, fetching a chair or making a drink for someone all promote happiness but may not strictly speaking be nursing activities.

Consequentialism pros and cons

When considering how helpful a consequentialist view of a situation might be we have to take heed of some of the pros and cons which apply to this form of normative ethics.

Some of the positive aspects of consequentialism include:

- It is neutral with respect to people involved; the moral calculus includes everyone concerned and treats them as equals.
- Consequentialism judges the ethicality of an action and not a person.
- Activity viewed from a consequentialist view is undertaken in order to achieve a predetermined goal.

For nursing, therefore, the application of consequentialism to what we do can be positive in that its neutrality means it is a good tool to use when considering the generation of local or national policy; it has its place in considering the allocation of resources and it strongly reflects the need for nurses to demonstrate leadership in the management of issues such as risk (as identified in the competencies at the start of the chapter).

The emphasis on the judgement of the action and not the person also reflects competency 2 in Domain 1, which talks about being *non-judgemental* and avoiding *assumptions*. The forward-looking nature of the consequentialist calculus reflects well the *outcome-focused* nature of the nursing process.

As well as all of the positives, there are a number of criticisms which apply to using utilitarianism as an ethical guide, including:

- It is difficult to make a calculation about the greatest good when emotional responses are involved – for example, if the issue being debated includes a family member.
- It is not possible to measure happiness objectively (or indeed, many alternative outcomes).
- It is not possible to know the exact amount of happiness an action might bring about.
- The time taken to undertake a utilitarian calculus could take so long that the event to which it is being applied may have passed.
- How do we account for difference of opinion about the benefit of outcomes?
- Consequentialism overlooks notions of **rights** and duties.

So consequentialism can be problematic for the nurse in that it is not easy to apply, takes an inordinate amount of time and, anyway, the exact outcomes we are supposed to maximise using the consequentialist calculus are not always well defined.

As a methodology for ethical decision making in nursing, consequentialist theories do have a place. What determines their usefulness is the ability within the given situation to account for all of the likely outcomes and the magnitude of the impact on the individuals involved.

Taking a broader view of the understanding of ethics in general, one of the positives of considering consequentialism as one of many methodologies and influences on ethical decision making is the fact that it provides a different lens through which to approach a scenario to almost all other approaches.

Non-consequentialism and rule-based theories

If consequentialist theories are about the outcome of an action, non-consequentialism is all about the action which brings about the consequences. Sometimes called **duty-based ethics** or **deontology**, this school of thought judges the morality of an action, or lack of action, in terms of the rules which should govern how we behave. The word deontology is derived from the Greek *deon*, which means duty. From the non-consequentialist perspective, it is not the outcome which matters; it is *what we do* that is important, regardless of result.

Non-consequentialism has its roots in Judeo-Christian theology and is perhaps reflective of the rules which appear in the Torah and the Bible, an example of which includes *Thou shalt not murder*. Immanuel Kant is perhaps the most famous deontologist. Kant (1785) believed that the only good actions were those which followed the *moral law*. Kant's moral law could be applied to, and by, all people in all situations. The moral law Kant refers to is absolute and applies in all situations regardless of the context and consequences. For example, lying is always wrong in this view even if it has detrimental consequences – this is primarily because we would not want lying to become the norm. So duty-based theories are about establishing ways of behaving which we all should follow at all times with no reference to the consequences.

Theory summary: Kant's rule of universality

Act only according to that maxim whereby you can, at the same time, will that it should become a universal law.

(Kant, 1785)

Meaning:

Always undertake actions which you wish would become the way people always behave in similar situations.

What Kant is getting at is the single and simple point that if we are to have rules of behaviour then all individuals must follow those rules because they are rational. He suggests that we ought to have rules about how to live and that these rules are the sort of thing any rational person would decide on through the application of reason. There is both simplicity to this view, because it is easier to follow rules, and a difficulty, in that it is not always clear what the rules are or when they apply – nor indeed what constitutes a rational being. Notably the view of **universality** expressed by Kant resounds with the viewpoint of many major world religions and is sometimes known as the **golden rule** or **ethic of reciprocity**.

Four principles approach

Over a number of years and in various editions of their book, Beauchamp and Childress (2012) have developed a duty-based theory of ethics: the **four principles approach**. This approach has proved to be very influential in western thinking about **moral dilemmas** and is widely taught and used in schools of both nursing and medicine, as well as other health-related disciplines. While these principles do not provide a complete overview of thought in the area of duty-based ethical theories, they provide a satisfactory tool for us to explore the nature of duty-based ethics and how they might apply to nursing practice.

The four principles of biomedical ethics

1   *Beneficence*
2   *Non-maleficence*
3   *Autonomy*
4   *Justice.*

(Beauchamp and Childress, 2012)

Beneficence

Beneficence is about *doing good*. In everyday language the word beneficence refers to any acts of kindness, benevolence and altruism; in ethical thought this concept is considered to include any activity which promotes the best interests of others (*Stanford Dictionary of Philosophy*, 2013). According to this principle healthcare professionals should always act in a manner which will be of greatest benefit to the patient in their care. On face value this is a principle all nurses would agree with and strive to achieve; there are some important questions which need to be asked about beneficence, however:

- What is a benefit to the patient?
- Who judges what a benefit is?
- What if the patient and the nurse disagree as to what is a benefit?
- Should this be a short-term gain or a long-term benefit?
- What about actions we do which cause immediate harm, even if they cause later benefit?

These are fundamental questions which can cause all manner of problems when trying to apply such principles in everyday nursing practice.

Activity 4.4	Critical thinking

Maureen's husband is not easily swayed in his view that taking her home to die would be the best course of action. Some of the staff agree that telling her what her diagnosis is would upset her. How should the ward team behave? In considering how to act, you should pay regard to rules of beneficence.

Activity 4.4 lays bare one of the problems with rule-based theories in that if one follows the rules then one should not lie; on the other hand, lying *might* promote the best interests of Maureen (be beneficent) in this scenario.

Non-maleficence

Non-maleficence is about *avoiding doing harm*. According to this rule, the nurse should always act in a manner which causes no harm to the patient. This appears to be a reasonable rule to abide by, but like beneficence, there are some issues with applying this in practice:

- What is harm?
- Who judges what harm is?
- What if the patient and the nurse disagree as to what is a harm?
- Does this apply to short-term or long-term harm?
- What about actions we do which cause immediate harm, even if they cause later benefit?

Activity 4.5	Critical thinking

The ward team has decided to overrule Maureen's husband and tell her what her diagnosis is. They argue that she is a competent adult and she has the right to know what is happening to her. The more senior members of the team say that lying to her will have negative consequences above and beyond those of withholding the truth. Do you think that telling Maureen her diagnosis is a good way to avoid doing harm? What other forms of harm might occur if she is not told?

It might appear that avoiding harm and doing good (non-maleficence and beneficence) are merely different sides of the same coin, that by doing good one is avoiding harm, but they are not the same thing. Johnstone (2009) makes the useful observation that there is a world of difference between the obligations not to kill someone (non-maleficence) and the duty to help someone in immediate danger (beneficence). What 'avoiding harm' requires is that we understand who we are harming and how and try to avoid doing this unless on balance it is necessary to achieve a 'good' which is of greater magnitude than the harm caused.

Autonomy

Autonomy is about having the *freedom to choose* a course of action; the word autonomy is derived from the Greek *auto* (self) and *nomos* (law). Autonomy requires the nurse always to take into account the choices of the patient. Respect for autonomy is a cornerstone of modern life, no more so than in the care setting, where people make decisions about what happens to them and their body.

The Mental Capacity Act (2005) recognises in law the right to autonomy and self-determination of the individual. There are five principles enshrined in the Act which demonstrate respect for autonomy:

(1) A person must be assumed to have capacity unless it is established that he lacks capacity.
(2) A person is not to be treated as unable to make a decision unless all practicable steps to help him to do so have been taken without success.
(3) A person is not to be treated as unable to make a decision merely because he makes an unwise decision.
(4) An act done, or decision made, under this Act for or on behalf of a person who lacks capacity must be done, or made, in his best interests.
(5) Before the act is done, or the decision is made, regard must be had to whether the purpose for which it is needed can be as effectively achieved in a way that is less restrictive of the person's rights and freedom of action.

Principles 1–3 establish in law what the ethical principle of autonomy seeks to do, that is generally accept people generally have the right to exercise choice, they should be given the facts they need to make a choice and that they are allowed to make what the professional may consider to be bad choices (The Stationery Office, 2005).

There are some tensions which arise for nurses who want to respect the choices that a patient makes when the choices do not appear to be in the best interests of the patient. We discuss autonomy in more detail in Chapter 6.

Activity 4.6   *Decision making*

In Maureen's case, there are options as to how and where she could experience her end-of-life care. The palliative care team argue that it is important that she is allowed to make these decisions for herself and telling her what her diagnosis and prognosis are is important as it respects and promotes her autonomy. Do you agree?

One of the biggest challenges which faces nurses in promoting the exercise of autonomy is the very nature of the care setting. All consumers of care are vulnerable regardless of who they are or why they are in the care setting. This vulnerability arises out of being ill, meeting care professionals who know the system and the language, perhaps being elderly or young. This vulnerability often deprives people of the ability to act truly autonomously – we will explore these issues in Chapter 6.

Justice

Classically we consider justice as referring to *being fair*. Fairness requires that we treat people in equal situations in an equal manner. This is, however, an incredibly difficult concept to get right. What do we mean by equal? Which people count? What exactly is fair?

Concept summary: veil of ignorance

In his classic book *A Theory of Justice*, Rawls (1999) refines the classic ethical thought experiment used to assess the justice of a given activity. In the 'veil of ignorance' experiment one has no knowledge of one's own position on a topic, nor of one's own leanings or place in society. The best rules for society are made by people agreeing on what these rules might be from behind this veil of ignorance, Rawls suggests. The beauty of this thought experiment is that there is some distribution of fairness because people are attempting to protect their own interests whilst being ignorant of what those interests might be.

Rawls' veil of ignorance experiment provides nurses with some ideas about what justice might look like in that, at the very least, it makes us ask the question: 'what if that were me or someone I love?' Nevertheless, justice is a hard concept to understand. Fry et al. (2011) provide a useful definition of two forms of justice. The first relates to *ethically correct allocation* (p. 111), where the distribution of some good is made on the basis of an ethical principle. They term the second form of justice the *narrow sense* (p. 111); this refers more to how the good (a service or resource, for example) is allocated according to some principle, which has to do with the allocation process itself (such as the greatest need or being the most deserving). On one definition, then, justice is itself an ethical principle and, on the other, it is a tool to enact other ethical principles.

Activity 4.7   *Decision making*

If we are to consider the justice of telling Maureen about her diagnosis, or not, we would have to consider what justice means for her case. Can we say she deserves to know what her diagnosis is and that it is the sort of action we ought to take in all such cases? Or is her husband correct in asserting her greater need is to be kept in the dark and to be allowed to die in ignorance of her condition? From the point of view of justice, what might be the right decision and why?

In Activity 4.7 justice can be considered as doing whatever the right thing is because that is what we always do and that makes it fair – so perhaps always telling the truth. Alternatively, it might be seen as a way of achieving the most right thing to do, which in this case might arguably be said to be avoiding doing harm (although it is not clear what course of action this might send us down). The third and perhaps hardest to achieve route is deciding what people like Maureen want in situations like this (treating people in equal situations in an equal manner). This might require that we gain an understanding of the sort of person Maureen is and use this to inform our decision making.

Scope

Beauchamp and Childress (2012) recognised that any ethical approach to decision making has to take account of the context within which it is applied as well as the situation to which it is being applied. To their four principles they therefore added the notion of scope. Scope applies to the fact that some *judgement* will need to be used in the application of the four principles.

The notion of scope is a practical response to the sorts of scenarios we have been looking at regarding whether to tell Maureen her diagnosis. In this case it is possible to justify both lying and not lying using any number of arguments. Scope allows flexibility within the process to ask pertinent questions (for example, about the decisions Maureen has taken about similar situations in the past) which might impact on the way in which we apply one of the four principles.

In the Maureen example, scope might lead us to ask other questions about Maureen's capacity to understand the prognosis; it might lead us to question the nature of her relationship with her husband or perhaps the manner in which he presents his argument.

Activity 4.8 — Critical thinking

On hearing that the team have decided to tell Maureen about her diagnosis, Maureen's husband comes to have a word with you. He tells you that Maureen has seen members of her family die from similar diseases and is not scared of death itself, but she has told him that if the same thing were to happen to her, she would not want to know about it. How might consideration of scope make you consider which, if any, of the four principles is the most important to apply in this situation?

In this iteration of the scenario what we have is both a potential clarifier (a reason to act in a specific way which identifies the important principle) as well as something which might serve to muddy our duty-based waters. In the first instance we can see how acting on what we are told are Maureen's express wishes will protect her *autonomy*, making this the most important of the principles; in the second we can see how lying might contribute to a general demise in beneficence and non-maleficence. What becomes clear, therefore, is that Beauchamp and Childress's *four principles plus scope* approach to ethical thinking is not as straightforward as it might appear.

Non-consequentialism pros and cons

There are many good aspects of duty-based theories of ethics, not least of which is the fact that all of the rules, the duties we must follow, apply to everyone equally. Non-consequentialists therefore treat people as **ends in themselves** rather than as a **means to an end**. This idea is attractive not only in general but to nurses in particular.

> ## Concept summary: 'ends in themselves' and 'means to an end'
>
> This is an important concept in ethical thinking for nurses as the Nursing and Midwifery Council (2015, p. 2) exhorts us to: *put the interests of people using or needing nursing or midwifery services first. You make their care and safety your main concern and make sure that their dignity is preserved*
>
> This important aspect of *The Code* recognises that we need to treat people as ends in themselves, that is, as beings capable of making their own decisions rather than as objects on which to practise our nursing (as a means to an end).
>
> We often talk ill of people who exploit others to get what they want with no regard for the effects of 'being used'. The idea of people as ends in themselves suggests a healthy respect for people, autonomy and the protection and promotion of dignity.

A further positive for duty-based theories is that people know where they are with rules. This means that not only do we know how to act, but we can also judge the actions of others by what they have done; there is no ambiguity. When individuals act out of duty, their intention to 'do their duty' is clear; this is in direct contrast to consequentialist actions where if the desired consequence is not achieved, people might, as we saw, claim 'that was not my intention'.

There are some recurring problems with non-consequentialist theories in that there may be conflicts between rules which makes it hard to decide which rule to follow in a given situation (as we saw with Maureen). This ambiguity might lead to inertia.

A further and major flaw of duty-based ethics lies in the fact that some actions, even though correct in themselves, can lead to outcomes which are very negative. Where negative consequences are anticipated it would seem unreasonable to ignore these for the sake of following a rule.

Virtue theory

In complete contrast to consequentialist and non-consequentialist theory, virtue theory is more concerned with *moral character*. The virtuous person does what is right and in the right way because that is what the virtuous person does. Unlike consequentialists, virtuous nurses do not seek to act to achieve a desired outcome and unlike duty theorists, they do not follow prescribed moral rule. Virtue theorists instead focus on the development of good habits of character; essentially the development of self, to become a *good person* (much like the development of self through guided reflection discussed in Chapters 1 and 2).

While consequentialist and non-consequentialist approaches to ethics both use the term virtue, they refer to this in the sense in which it applies to the decision of the individual to follow the rules of that particular school of ethical thought. For the utilitarian and deontologist, then, ethicality is about applying and sticking to the rules which govern their approach to ethics. In virtue theory, the whole basis of decision making is completely different: virtuous people act in a certain way because they understand what is important in how human life is to be led. As Hodkinson (2008, p. 248) points out: *Strong virtue ethics is a single theory which needs no supplementation from other ethical frameworks.*

This is quite confusing on the one level. How can we generate a theory which appears to lead the individual user to different conclusions in similar and subtly different circumstances, or indeed two virtue theorists in the same circumstance?

Activity 4.9 *Critical thinking*

Maureen's husband asks if he might discuss his decision about not letting her know her diagnosis. He says he is somewhat confused by the reaction of the staff as some seem to support him and others do not. He wonders if he is doing the right thing by Maureen. You are unsure what you think about the situation, but you are clear about what is important in human relationships. As a virtuous nurse, what questions might help you to understand better how to advise and support Maureen and her husband?

The answers to Activity 4.9 lie in the understanding of people and most especially around what is important in being human. Maureen's husband is looking for the right thing to do, not from the point of view of duty or consequences, but what is right for Maureen as a human being. These notions point us in the direction from which virtue theory emanates.

Concept summary: the philosophical basis of virtue theory

Virtue theory has its roots in ancient Greek philosophy where the *ethical being* exercised a number of interconnected concepts, the three most important of which are:

1. *Arete:* this is about excellence (or perhaps even virtue itself).
2. *Phronesis:* this is practical understanding or moral wisdom (the kind of intrinsic knowing).
3. *Eudaimonia:* human flourishing. This concerns living a fulfilled life in which fulfilment comes from attaining some of the human goods such as integrity and dignity and living a life which is 'virtuous'.

There is much to be said for the translation of these concepts into the moral life of the nurse. Clearly, as a practical profession, nursing lends itself to ethical theories which value practicality – the sort of moral wisdom which can emerge from practice, reflection and working with others is a theme which runs throughout this book (see especially Chapter 2). What is unclear is exactly what practical wisdom looks like and how it can be said to operate in nursing; that said, the fact that it is hard to identify or measure empirically (see Chapter 8) does not mean that there is not a strong shared intuition among nurses as to what is the right thing to do in many situations (Woodard Leners, 1992). Indeed, Aristotle (translated by Thompson, 1976) held that the right, virtuous action is that which is the best practically; by 'best' he meant for the person to flourish (see below). For Aristotle this was the only moral consideration.

If nursing is about achieving excellence in care then there is something also to be said for consideration of excellence within an ethical theory which relates to nursing. On a superficial level this might suggest that achieving excellence in care is the ethical thing to do; on a more philosophical level excellence is about achieving all we can as humans and for humans, excellence is in itself the virtue. Adams (2006) presents a clear and helpful exposition on what virtue theory might mean; his explanation of excellence and its relationship to virtue is especially helpful. Adams sees virtue as excellence; he regards excellence as *being for the good*. Furthermore he regards *being for the good* as having the disposition (nature or character) which strives for excellence in *action, desire, emotion or feeling* (p. 17). This explanation suggests that the ethical nurse is ethical by character and perhaps that character is arrived at through choice.

There is an appeal to this as a theory of ethics since, unlike consequentialism and non-consequentialism, it is the nature of the person which drives the decision making and not the decision-making process itself. This means we are not distracted by trying to fit a model to a scenario, but rather the virtuous nurse just knows what the best thing to do is.

The third concept, flourishing, has an appeal to the practice of nursing, the end goal of which is to achieve the wellbeing (flourishing) of those we care for. Again there is a superficial appeal which perhaps comes from the connectedness of this idea to physical and perhaps mental flourishing. Indeed, one of the default diagnoses sometimes seen in hospital where a patient has perhaps just given up is 'failure to thrive'; that is another way of saying the patient is no longer flourishing. But this is too tenuous a link to help virtue theory appeal to the conscientious nurse and does not relate to the notion that it is through flourishing as a nurse that one might achieve virtue. In Aristotle's view, flourishing is achieved through integrity in thought and action. Conversely we fail to flourish as nurses when we allow things to happen around us that we know are wrong, something we identified in Chapter 1 as *moral stress*.

Armstrong (2006) suggests four good reasons why nurses might adopt virtue theory as a guide to action, although (like all virtue theorists) he also points out we cannot divorce who we are in work from who we are outside.

Merits of virtue ethics in nursing

1. *It reflects the sort of words and language nurses use in their daily practice, e.g. care, well and fair.*
2. *It emphasises the role of emotion in the working and ethical lives of nurses.*
3. *It recognises the need to exercise judgement in making decisions of a moral nature given the multiple context of care in which nurses work.*
4. *It recognises the place of role models in the development of the ethically active nurse.*

(Adapted from Armstrong, 2006)

Armstrong also usefully points out that virtue theory, unlike consequentialism and non-consequentialism, which are quite set and unbending, can be said to be *context-dependent, relational, and particularist* (Armstrong, 2006, p. 121).

One of the biggest problematic issues with virtue theory is that it is not entirely intuitive. That is to say, one has to undertake some work, thinking and reflecting, in order to start to understand what it means and how it applies to nursing practice. This issue is linked to the second issue in that, because there are no rules to follow as such, it is quite difficult to teach and learn virtue and it is perhaps best thought of as a way of being which the nurse grows into. This leads us to the final problem with virtue theory in that it is hard to know when we have reached the state of being virtuous enough to allow virtue to drive our ethical decision making.

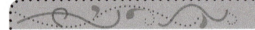

Chapter summary

This chapter has introduced you to some of the main ethical and philosophical ideas which inform ethical decision making in the clinical setting. Through the use of some clinical scenarios we have seen that sometimes the theories can complement each other and in other scenarios they might be directly opposed. In this chapter we have explored the three predominant theories which inform normative ethics in the UK today: consequentialism, non-consequentialism (deontology) and virtue theory.

We have seen that consequentialism and non-consequentialism guide action through the application of rules which are applied to a situation in order to get an answer to an ethical issue. We have seen that, in direct contrast to the other two theories, virtue theory does not start from the application of rules but of understanding what is important in human interactions.

Activities: brief outline answers

Activity 4.1 Decision making

Using Bentham's utilitarian calculus it is hard to say what the outcome of lying to Maureen might be. Certainly there may be a short-term reduction in her mental pain by not knowing and this may give her more pleasure and perhaps even her husband on one level – together this could amount to a lot of pleasure. On the other hand her husband has the pain and effort of keeping the truth from her; she may detect something is not right and have to contend with the pain of being lied to and the pain of guessing she is dying, and trying to pretend she does not know. The hospital staff will not gain pleasure by telling Maureen the truth, but they will at least be spared the pain of having to lie if they tell her about her condition. Using act utilitarianism can therefore be very confusing.

Activity 4.2 Decision making

The calculation which needs to be made here is a little more complex. What rule utilitarianism allows, that act utilitarianism does not, is some consideration of the nature of pleasure and pain as well as the meaning of the decision within the context of broader society. So in this case, as well as the issues identified in the answer to Activity 4.1, we might consider the negative effects on society of allowing lies to be told to competent patients; the lack of respect for individuals which arises from allowing others to make decisions about them; the impact of not doing what the hospital staff considers right. Rule utilitarianism, while remaining complex and working with equations which are by no means certain, does have the advantage of taking a broader view of what an outcome might be and therefore is perhaps not as difficult to work with as act utilitarianism.

Activity 4.4 Critical thinking

It is difficult to know what doing good means in this scenario. On the one hand, always acting according to the sort of rule which might suggest doing good requires us always to tell the truth. This type of decision has to be made regardless of the consequences and relates to the behaviour itself – which perhaps seems a little harsh in certain circumstances. Conversely, telling the truth suggests that the staff are also showing respect for Maureen as a competent and capable individual and, surely, this ought to be one of the universal rules.

Activity 4.5 Critical thinking

As in Activity 4.4, it is hard to know what we mean by harm here. If we lie to Maureen then we have done harm by failing to follow our rule of not lying, but if we take the husband's view we might minimise the harm done (which is perhaps a more consequentialist approach). But also by lying to Maureen there is the real danger we will harm her relationship with us as professionals – and with her husband – as she will work things out for herself.

Activity 4.6 Decision making

Respecting autonomy generally means allowing people to make decisions about things which affect them. In an ideal world we would already know what sort of decision patients would make and follow their predetermined plan. The question here is: do we believe it is respectful of autonomy to keep the truth from someone or are we treating Maureen with a lack of respect? Perhaps her husband knows her better and in fact she would choose not to know and therefore not telling her the truth is in this case more in keeping with respecting her autonomy.

Activity 4.7 Decision making

With respect to justice it is hard to see how this might apply to Maureen's scenario. What we really need to consider is how we might normally act in these situations. In this respect, rather than being a tool in itself, justice is a guide to how we might apply the other ethical tools (in this case, beneficence, non-maleficence and autonomy) in other broadly similar situations. What precedent do we want to create which might become the rule for future scenarios; do we want to lie or tell the truth?

Activity 4.8 Critical thinking

As it is seen in operation here, scope might mean that we have to adapt our understanding of what is the usual 'right thing to do' and consider the circumstances which are operating here. If Maureen has been the sort of person who never wants to hear about her illnesses, has never wanted to discuss the details of surgery and has told her husband to hide any such facts from her in the future, then perhaps this serves to turn on their head our preconceptions about doing good, avoiding harm and justice. This conscious decision not to know might be considered to be a reasonable exercise of Maureen's autonomy and perhaps autonomy is more important than any of the other principles in this case? Of course, if we were talking about an impact on other people, then justice might be more important or perhaps avoiding harm, so scope is very situational and requires considerable thought before it is applied.

Activity 4.9 Critical thinking

There is no doubt the usual response to this sort of scenario is to say that the team will not lie to Maureen. This scenario is, however, quite a difficult one to unpack. The virtuous nurse understands that the devil is in the detail with such dilemmas and that it is important to discuss with Maureen's husband in some depth their relationship, not only to inform the decision which is eventually made but also to be able to support him through it. The virtuous nurse will understand that the decision must be congruent with who Maureen is, the decisions she has made in the past and what she has told her family she wants. They will understand that this is about the person and the situation rather than the application of a school of ethical thought.

Further reading

Armstrong, AE (2006) Towards a strong virtue ethics for nursing practice. *Nursing Philosophy*, 7(3): 110–124.
A clear argument in favour of virtue ethics in nursing.

Buka, P (2014) *Patients' Rights, Law and Ethics for Nurses*, 2nd edn. London: CRC.
See especially Chapters 1 and 2.

Useful websites

www.surrey.ac.uk/fhms/research/centres/ICE/resources/index.htm
A good list of resources about healthcare and nursing ethics

Chapter 5
Rights

Peter Ellis

NMC Standards for Pre-registration Nursing Education

This chapter will address the following competencies:

Domain 1: Professional values

3. All nurses must support and promote the health, wellbeing, rights and dignity of people, groups, communities and populations. These include people whose lives are affected by ill health, disability, ageing, death and dying. Nurses must understand how these activities influence public health.

Domain 2: Communication and interpersonal skills

4. All nurses must recognise when people are anxious or in distress and respond effectively, using therapeutic principles, to promote their wellbeing, manage personal safety and resolve conflict. They must use effective communication strategies and negotiation techniques to achieve best outcomes, respecting the dignity and human rights of all concerned. They must know when to consult a third party and how to make referrals for advocacy, mediation or arbitration.

8. All nurses must respect individual rights to confidentiality and keep information secure and confidential in accordance with the law and relevant ethical and regulatory frameworks, taking account of local protocols. They must also actively share personal information with others when the interests of safety and protection override the need for confidentiality.

Domain 4: Leadership, management and team working

4. All nurses must be self-aware and recognise how their own values, principles and assumptions may affect their practice. They must maintain their own personal and professional development, learning from experience, through supervision, feedback, reflection and evaluation.

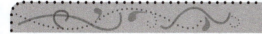

NMC Essential Skills Clusters

This chapter will address the following ESCs:

Care, compassion and communication

Patients/clients can trust a newly registered graduate nurse to:

2. Engage in person centred care empowering people to make choices about how their needs are met when they are unable to meet them for themselves.

(continued)

continued . . .

3. Respect them as individuals and strive to help them preserve their dignity at all times.
6. Engage therapeutically and actively listen to their needs and concerns, responding using skills that are helpful, providing information that is clear, accurate, meaningful and free from jargon.
7. Protect and keep as confidential all information relating to them.
8. Gain their consent based on sound understanding and informed choice prior to any intervention and that their rights in decision making and consent will be respected and upheld.

Cluster: Organisational aspects of care
Patients/clients can trust a newly registered graduate nurse to:
11. Safeguard children and adults from vulnerable situations and support and protect them from harm.
14. Be an autonomous and confident member of the multidisciplinary or multiagency team and to inspire confidence in others.
18. Enhance the safety of service users and identify and actively manage risk and uncertainty in relation to people, the environment, self and others.

Chapter aims

After reading this chapter you will be able to:

- critically discuss the nature of rights;
- understand how you might promote and protect the rights of people in your care;
- identify what considerations might give rise to rights;
- consider why the right to confidentiality is so important in healthcare settings.

Introduction

The language of rights is pervasive in modern society. It is very common to hear phrases such as 'I have a right to … ', 'that is my right' or 'I know my rights'. Most certainly there are a whole host of rights which nurses need to be aware of in the delivery of care, including normal human rights (the sort of thing captured in the European Declaration of Human Rights), as well as special rights (which are conferred upon patients by virtue of the fact they are in our care at any given point in time).

The language of rights can often be quite confusing. How rights work, or as philosophers say 'operate', is somewhat mysterious. Where rights come from and who is entitled to hold a given right are not always immediately apparent. What should be done when one right contradicts another right (when rights conflict) is a source of regular tension in the clinical setting.

This chapter is slightly different to most of the other chapters, as within it we will address some of the issues raised above as well as proposing a basis for where rights in healthcare might come from as well as how they might *operate*.

For the purposes of this chapter especially, we will use the term *rights* to mean something quite specific. In this context, the word rights will not denote the difference between *rights* and *wrongs*, as in *good* and *bad*. Instead this chapter seeks to identify rights as ethical tools which may be used to inform our ethical decision making in practice. Most especially we will consider what rights mean for us in terms of how they inform nursing activity and healthcare provision on a wider scale. Rights deserve a chapter all to themselves as they are very special ethically and morally and, given what we will see in this chapter, they might be used to overrule other ethical considerations in some circumstances. This ability to '**trump**' other ethical considerations such as consequentialism or duties (Dworkin, 1992) makes them different to all other approaches to ethics and therefore a tool for ethical decision making which nurses should understand.

One of the corollaries of rights are duties. As part of the process of expanding on what rights are and why they are important we will also examine the duty of the nurse to maintain confidentiality as well as the notion of duty of care.

What are rights?

The simplest way of thinking about rights is to consider when people call upon (evoke) them. People often claim a right as a means of getting something they want or need, but this cannot provide a sufficient answer. As with all ethical ideas and concepts, rights arise only in the context of society. Essentially rights exist to protect the individual from unreasonable and unwanted interference. In this respect the right belongs to the individual and is not part of any calculation (as we saw in consequentialism) or any requirement to follow some rule (as we saw with non-consequentialism).

Concept summary: the function of rights

The important idea to grasp about rights lies in the sentence above, which says: *rights exist to protect the individual from unreasonable and unwanted interference*. At first glance this looks like a simple concept, but it lays bare some challenges: if rights protect the individual, should society suffer as a result? What happens when more than one person claims a right and they oppose each other? The answer to this lies in considering the terms unreasonable and unwanted (see case study below). Unreasonable suggests interference which has no legitimate ethical basis; this suggests quite strongly there are actions which involve interfering with the life of another person and these actions are both reasonable and have a legitimate ethical basis. Examples where interference is reasonable might include the deprivation of liberty as it applies to a person with advanced dementia or preventing someone with mental illness from harming others (see the Mental Capacity Act, 2005; the Stationery Office, 2005).

> ## Case study: unwarranted and unwanted interference
>
> *Ms B was left a tetraplegic by a haemorrhage into her cervical spine. She made a request to her treating doctors to stop her ventilation and to allow her to die. The doctors refused and had her competence assessed. The initial assessment found her not to be competent to make decisions, but a subsequent assessment ruled she was. Despite her competence, doctors treating her refused her request and so Ms B went to court in order to compel the doctors to stop her ventilation. In 2002 the High Court ruled her request was valid and treatment was stopped. The court ruling had pointed to the fact that people have the right to decide what happens to them regardless of the consequences and that grave consequences for the individual are not indicative of incompetence (Slowther, 2002).*
>
> *Ms B clearly did not wish to be ventilated and the ruling established that the healthcare professionals had no right to impose it on her; in this respect the treatment was both unwanted and unreasonable and the exercise of Ms B's right to decide what happened to her body protected her from ongoing treatment.*

At first glance then rights are very individualistic; they relate to a person and have little to do with anyone else. This idea is mostly correct as rights exist purely to operate as protection for individuals (although many people can lay claim to the same right at the same time). The operation of some rights does have meaning for other individuals, since one person's right might be another person's duty, but this is not always the case, as we shall see.

So rights operate on more than one level and it is important therefore that we establish what this means for nurses, and the actions we must undertake. Before we look at how rights might operate and what this means for nurses, it is worth thinking about where rights might come from and what exactly it is about the person which they seek to protect.

Think of it like this: rights do not grow on trees. They have some legal, philosophical and ethical basis (Ellis, 2012); it is this basis which not only establishes their existence, but also their scope (how widely they apply), who they apply to and what they require of others in the way of doing something or leaving someone alone. In the next part of the chapter we will consider where various forms of rights come from and therefore the extent to which they might operate in nursing and healthcare in general.

The basis of rights

If we are to claim to have rights, or indeed if our patients are to claim to have rights, then it is important not only that we know what these rights are and how they operate, but also that we have some idea what the basis for these rights might be.

For the purposes of this book we will consider three forms of rights: legal rights, special rights and human rights. The most difficult of these to comprehend are human rights and so we will examine these last. In terms of priming your thinking for the rest of the chapter, it is important here to state that, in the context of this book, human rights are not going to be considered in relation to the European Convention on Human Rights and the ensuing Human Rights Act and attendant legislation. Instead in this chapter the Human Rights Act will be considered as a legal right, with human rights belonging to all humans regardless of the existence of laws.

Legal rights

Legal rights are the rights that belong to us all as citizens of a country, or indeed of the world, when these rights are either laid out in statute or have evolved in **case law**. Legal rights only operate in the jurisdiction of the law-making body. So, for example, laws which are in place in the UK only relate to the UK and do not apply in France. On the other hand, European Union laws apply throughout those countries which are members of the European Union. International law is completely different as on the whole it applies only to the relationships between sovereign states and does not apply to individuals.

Activity 5.1 — Reflection

Think about all the things which you have a legal right to claim because you live in this country. What rights have you asserted today just by virtue of being a citizen?

There are some possible answers to all activities at the end of the chapter, unless otherwise indicated.

We are so used to asserting our rights in the UK that it is easy to forget just how many we have and what they give us in the way of different forms of freedoms.

As nurses operating within a legislated healthcare system, legal rights play an important part in our day-to-day lives, since our fellow citizens have a legally conferred and protected right to expect a certain standard of care. That said, this book is an ethics textbook and so we will continue to examine rights within healthcare from a more ethical perspective.

Special rights

Special rights are of considerable interest to nurses and care providers in general because special rights arise out of the special obligations we agree to take on in our position as care givers.

Special rights are not like other rights as they are not necessarily universal – that is, they do not apply to all human beings equally. While the sort of special rights our patients have has a basis in law, or at least in our nursing code of conduct, they do not apply to everyone all at the same time.

Special rights are created when two people, or groups of people, enter into a relationship in which they both accept the right and the corresponding duties which go with that right. For example, in the UK the *right to healthcare* arises out of the special relationship the citizens have with the state; the duty of the state to provide healthcare (in the form of the National Health Service (NHS)) comes about because we as citizens have agreed it should exist and many of us contribute to its existence through the payment of taxes and national insurance.

So the right to healthcare in the UK is not the same thing as the *right to health*. The right to healthcare has a particular meaning which is tied up in the contract between the state, the care providers and the citizens of the state. The right to healthcare in the UK extends to citizens of the UK, not because they are human per se, but because they belong to a group of people with whom the government has a special relationship – its citizens.

Activity 5.2   *Critical thinking*

What does the existence of the right to healthcare mean in terms of providing care to people who are not part of the special relationship? Do you think this arrangement has other ethical and moral dimensions not captured in the preceding definition? How do you feel about the relationship between being a citizen and the right to access healthcare in a particular setting?

The special relationship which gives rise to rights in the healthcare setting is born out of the fact that as nurses we agree to provide care. As part of the relationship between the nurse and the patient, society agrees to pay nurses to provide care and it affords nurses a certain status. In return for being recognised as professionals and being paid a professional salary by society, nurses accept a duty of care.

What this duty of care entails is not easily defined. Some commentators believe this duty is to all people, and ideally it would be. More realistically, however, the duty extends to patients and patients are defined not only by need but also by their entitlement to care – although this is not something we worry about in the emergency care scenario – it is, as we saw above, a reality of the care setting.

Gracia (2011, p. 92) makes the interesting, and somewhat challenging, observation: *Our duty is always the same, to do the best.* What the *best* means is open to some interpretation, but who gets to define the best is clear: it is the patient – we will pick up on this idea a little later when we explore best interests.

Human rights

These are the most conceptual, but perhaps the most pervasive, of the rights we will discuss in this chapter. To some extent, for us as nurses human rights are superseded by special rights. Special rights are more important for us as nurses as they relate directly to what we do on a day-to-day basis and have a direct bearing on our professional lives. Regardless of this, however, the argument for the basis of human rights which we will advance in this section of the chapter is potentially very informative for us in practice and is worth considerable thought.

Many of the discussions about rights start with trying to identify what it is that the right is trying to protect the individual from. On the grand scale this is, as we discussed earlier, unwanted interference by the state.

Concept summary: the individual and the greater good

If society is formed to make our lives better, then one of the purposes of society is to improve the lot of as many people as possible within the resources available. Taking this notion at face value then, the state might say that people who contribute the most to society are more valuable than those who contribute the least. What then stops us as a society from killing those who contribute nothing or only take from society because surely getting rid of these people would advance the greater good? History is littered with examples of societies doing just this. For example, the Nazis killed people with learning disabilities because they were considered 'useless mouths', i.e. people who needed feeding but who contributed nothing to society. In the face of this sort of understanding of society, the individual and what is good for the individual are inconsequential and what is good for the many is what we should strive to achieve. Human rights provide one powerful counterbalance to this utilitarian view in that they seek to protect the individual human from the *greater good.*

As societies have developed, we have come to understand there is intrinsic value in all human beings and, while we might want to advance the good of the group, we cannot do this at the expense of some individuals. Philosophically then, we need something to protect the individual from considerations of the greater good, as laid out in the concept box above, and this something needs to be extensive and powerful enough not to be affected by changes in society or other elements of the law. This is where human rights come in.

Activity 5.3   *Research and finding out*

The United Nations adopted the Universal Declaration of Human Rights in 1948; find the text for this at: **www.un.org/en/documents/udhr** and reflect on what this means for you as a global citizen, wherever it is that you are reading this book. You might like to consider also how the many rights identified in this Declaration are demonstrated on a day-to-day basis in your life and what freedoms you enjoy as a result. Also consider what the Declaration requires of you as a person and a nurse.

As this answer is based on your own observations, there is no outline answer at the end of the chapter.

What is clear on reading the Universal Declaration of Human Rights is that it is intended to apply to all people at all times and in all places. This idea establishes the universality (that is, the comprehensiveness) of the ideas contained within it. Such rights and freedoms therefore apply equally to a person whether s/he is experiencing an episode of care or not.

So we have established there are some universal human rights, but this leaves us with an important question whose answer perhaps helps us to establish how and why we might allow human rights to guide what we do in the care setting. That question is: what is it about the individual human which is important enough to deserve the protection of rights?

Activity 5.4   *Reflection*

One way we can see the importance of human rights is to reflect on recent issues in the news which might suggest that individuals and societies may not fully live up to the ideals expressed within the Declaration. Look at the media and reflect upon the variety of issues in the news which show human rights being ignored or violated. Using some of the ideas contained in this chapter, reflect upon the value of rights as a means of protecting people – this need not be a healthcare-related issue.

As this answer is based on your own observations, there is no outline answer at the end of the chapter.

In answering this question we might start to glimpse something of the nature of how and why rights are important considerations in the healthcare setting as well as how we might usefully be informed by them in our activities as nurses. While there are many theories as to what the basis of rights might be (see Further Reading for a guide to some of these), in this book we will explore only one: the idea of interests.

Interests

In this section we will explore how interests might provide a basis for the granting of rights. The reason we have chosen interests over any of the other potential forms of justification is because they make intuitive and experiential sense to nurses who are familiar with terms such as 'in the patient's best interests'.

What then does it mean to have interests? And more specifically, what is it about interests which *might* deserve the protection of rights? The argument being put forward here is not that interests are necessarily the only basis for conferring rights on someone or something, but merely that interests provide us with one plausible reason to think that something which possesses interests might deserve the protection of rights. This argument also does not suggest that we have a right to every interest we have; if this were the case then we would all have the right to be healthy, wealthy and wise!

In the philosophical literature, interests appear to take one of two forms: those interests which are *physical* in nature and those which are *mental* or perhaps even *spiritual*. It is worth considering both forms of interests here so that we can start to understand what it is about interests, and best interests, which might deserve the protection of rights.

One of the arguments in Chapter 1 suggested that society, and more especially ethical behaviour, could quite conceivably have resulted from our need as a species to escape the *short, uncomfortable and brutal* natural state of being (Hobbes, edited by Tuck, 1991). Clearly living a life which is longer, comfortable and free of brutality might count as something which is in our best interests as humans and therefore might provide some clues as to what exactly does deserve the protection of rights.

Physical best interests are quite easy to understand as they arise from experiences which are common not only to humans but to many animals as well. We are all interested in the avoidance of pain, hunger and extremes of temperature. These are simple ideas and on some level they might reasonably expect the protection of rights. We can see this sort of thing in action not only in the human world, but also in respect to animal welfare. Singer (1986) in his classic text helps ground this argument as he points out that a stone cannot have interests because nothing we can do will harm a stone and therefore a stone is not the sort of thing we might expect to have rights. The logical corollary of this idea might conceivably be therefore that things which can experience physical sensation might deserve the protection of rights.

If rights existed only to protect us, and animals, from these negative physical experiences then could such rights claim to be human rights? What about people who are unconscious, the unborn, people with physical and/or mental impairment who may not experience sensations in the way the majority of us do? Do these people not deserve the protection of rights? If they do, and there seems to be a majority consensus that this is the case, then there has to be something more about being human which is deserving of the protection of human rights.

Clearly there is possibly something more about being human (see the arguments about abortion set out in Chapter 7) which suggests, to most people, that there is something special about us as a species and which therefore affords us the protection of rights which is not usually associated with other forms of animal life. The question is therefore: what is this specialness, this uniqueness, if indeed there is anything, which separates humans from other species in this respect?

If we stick to the language of interests we might find one potential answer. The point here is that there are other ways of explaining the importance of humans, and indeed other higher life forms, but we will follow the reasoning about interests through because it fits what nurses do. We commonly state in practice that we are doing this because it is in the 'patient's best interests', but if it does not just relate to physical things, what does this notion of best interests refer to?

> ## Concept summary: what it means to have interests
>
> Interests in the sense meant here refer to two distinct ideas. The first is the physical sense of interests, about the things which impact our physical sense. Dworkin (1993) identifies these as **experiential interests** as they relate directly to experiences. Dworkin (1993) further identifies a second form of interests. He calls these **critical interests**; these interests relate to issues of human judgement and the intrinsic worth of human life. They relate perhaps to issues around how people choose to lead their life (congruence – see Chapter 1) and might include ideas such as personal reputation (Levenbook, 1984) and perhaps dignity (Ellis, 1996).

In the care setting we make decisions which affect people all of the time. Some of these decisions are directly related to the best thing to do for individuals in relation to their ongoing care, while other decisions are about them as people. It is this distinction, between decisions about patients' care as opposed to those about them as people, which Benjamin and Curtis (2010) call *medical decisions in the technical sense* (p. 14) and *medical decisions in the contextual sense* (p. 15). In the technical, perhaps physical, sense, it is clear that decisions should be made based on the best available evidence which reflects good practice. Clearly the best interests here relate to the best medical and physical interests of the individual – what Dworkin (1993) called experiential interests.

It is in considering the other of Benjamin and Curtis's (2010) medical decision-making modes, *contextual*, that we start to see the place of best interests as a human condition starting to emerge. These contextual issues occur in nursing on a daily basis and may include matters of life and death (as we explore in Chapter 7); personal preference and the exercise of autonomy (as we explore in Chapter 6) and the exercise of values and personal and professional judgement. These decisions are not made with the benefit of medical or technical expertise and, as Benjamin and Curtis (2010, p. 15) point out, medical decisions in the contextual sense *will often turn on questions of value, and … the physician's technical expertise does not make him or her an expert on conflicts of value.*

Scenario: best interests

Gordon is in his mid-50s and has rapidly advancing multiple sclerosis. As a consequence of the illness Gordon falls a lot, struggles to feed himself and it is increasingly difficult to communicate with him. It is clear that Gordon's partner Nicola is struggling to care for him as each time you visit the house alone as part of your community placement he appears more unkempt and has bruises sustained in recent falls. You are very conflicted about what to do as you feel Gordon needs more help but he has told you he does not want you interfering and telling the district nurses about his recent falls as he is quite happy with the way things are.

(continued)

continued . . .

> *The conflict for the nurse lies in having the desire to serve Gordon's best interests in the technical sense while also respecting and wishing to protect his right to exercise his freedom to pursue what he regards as being in his best interest (in the contextual sense).*

What this scenario demonstrates takes us back to the start of the chapter and the discussion about what the word 'right' means. Clearly there are two right (correct/ethical) things to do here and so, as healthcare professionals, we are on the horns of a dilemma (see Chapter 7). The first right thing to do is to provide the care that we feel Gordon needs; the second right thing to do is to respect Gordon's and Nicola's wishes for independence. Possibly in cases such as this the ethical thing to do is to allow consideration of Gordon's *rights* to guide our decision making.

Activity 5.5   *Decision making*

Consider Gordon's case as laid out in the previous scenario. Using what you have learnt so far about right and wrong, rights and interests, think about what you might do if faced with a similar situation in practice. What might Gordon's situation require you to do and whose help might you call upon in order to help you decide what to do?

Scenarios such as this one point to the issue which often generates the ethical questions – the different ways in which people see the world. What is clear from this example is that, while Gordon's and Nicola's decision may be a bad one in the purely technical sense, on a personal level it may be right. It is the defence of the individual's right to make such decisions based on what s/he considers to be in his or her best interests which might provide a justifiable reason for the creation of rights.

As we see here, while interference from others may not be undertaken with bad intent, it could, at least in Gordon's eyes, be seen as unwanted. His right to ask for his situation to be kept secret may not be something a student nurse can grant but his right to turn down offers of further help appears reasonable.

There is a counter argument to this view which may be increasingly important as the population grows older and diseases of ageing such as dementia become more prevalent. Dresser (2010) questions the value of drawing a distinction between experiential and critical interests as many people do not or cannot do this. She gives the example of someone with dementia who could suffer experientially when a decision supported by the critical best interests is made even though they, as an individual, may no longer care about that critical interest.

Activity 5.6	Decision making

Consider Gordon's case as laid out in the previous scenario but in this activity replace multiple sclerosis with advanced dementia. Would it still be OK to allow Gordon to stay with Nicola if he is falling, bruised and not eating properly? Would it be alright to leave him in the care of Nicola if this had been what he had said he wanted to happen before his dementia became advanced?

What these activities point to is the individual nature of interests and therefore the individual operationalisation of the rights which serve to protect them. Of course, if people have the right to choose their own rights and how these operate, this would lead to chaos as some people will make choices which are self-centred and demand a lot of others. It is worth therefore considering how rights might operate and what this means for us not only as nurses but also as people.

How rights operate

One way in which we can illustrate how rights work is to consider how some of these rights operate in practice. This will include considering not only the nature of the right, but also the way in which the right might operate when it is in conflict with the rights, and perhaps duties, of other individuals. Clearly, as a concept, rights, which exist to protect the individual from unwarranted interference, cannot operate in such a way as to impose unwarranted interference on others!

Hart (1992) defines having rights as having a moral justification for limiting how other people should act. What this means in practice is, however, quite unclear.

Concept summary: what having a right means

Hohfeld (1919) provides what is widely viewed as the first and best overview of what 'x has a right to y' means:

- x is at **liberty** to do y (or at least under no duty not to).
- x has a **claim** that others shall not interfere with his or her achieving y (negative claim) or that others should help him or her to achieve y (positive claim).
- x has the power to change the form of the existing rights (e.g. to release someone from an obligation).
- x has an **immunity** so no one can change the form of right x has.

What these different classifications of rights demonstrate is that there are three elements at play: the *person with the right*, the *nature* (or strength) of the right and *what the right requires* of others. For instance, a liberty right demonstrates that, while someone may be at liberty to do something, no one else is under any obligation to help that person do it. In contrast, where there is a positive claim right, the individual can expect someone else (someone who holds the corresponding duty) to help him or her.

So when someone claims a right, or when we are considering our own rights and those of others, we really need to define what exactly we mean. This is important for two reasons: first, it defines what is required from us as nurses in the way of action or inaction and second, it gives us a mechanism to judge between rights when more than one right is claimed in a situation.

One complication here is that in situations which involve people there will often be more than one person claiming a right. The question for us, looking at the ethics of the situation, is whose claim to have their right respected is the strongest? Or indeed, if there is a person claiming a right but the impact on others will be great, should we uphold the right?

Dworkin (1987) makes some useful observations about rights which help us to consider these questions. Dworkin regards rights as tools for achieving liberties which help establish and maintain equality. In Dworkin's view rights exist only to protect the individual from consideration of general welfare, but, and this is an important but, when the consideration of general welfare is high (as for example in protecting the public from an individual who is severely mentally ill and a danger to others) the strength of the right is diminished.

In the next section we will explore the idea of the right to expect confidentiality in the nurse–patient/healthcare professional–patient relationship and use this discussion to help unpack how rights may or may not be said to operate in the healthcare setting.

The right to confidentiality

The right to confidentiality is one of the pillars of modern healthcare provision. We protect people's confidences both as a mark of respect for them as autonomous individuals and also because they have a positive legal and special claim right against us as healthcare professionals which requires this. This special claim right arises out of the fact that this is what we agree to do as we enter the profession and therefore the public expect us to honour this obligation.

Confidentiality requires that we as nurses do not divulge information about a patient's illnesses, life or family unless the patient has given us express permission to do so. We also do not divulge information to other people, including those the patient has identified to the team we can talk to, unless we have established their identity.

....

Case study: inadvertent breach of confidentiality

In late 2012 the Duchess of Cambridge was admitted to the King Edward VII hospital, London, with complications relating to her pregnancy. Two Australian DJs phoned the hospital, pretending to be members of the royal family, and were put through to the ward caring for the Duchess. A member of the nursing staff on the ward was taken in by the prank and passed some details of the Duchess's condition to the DJs over the phone. There was a furore in the immediate aftermath of the prank, with hospital chiefs, the Care Quality Commission and the Nursing and Midwifery Council all taking positions critical of the hospital staff involved. Tragically, some days after the event, one of the nurses involved, Jacintha Saldanha, took her own life.

....

This unfortunate incident points out just how seriously the staff involved took the incident. While no one was physically harmed, damage had been done to the Duchess of Cambridge as a consequence of making her medical details known to people who had no right to know them.

But does this mean that all patients at all times and in all situations have an absolute blanket claim over how we as nurses should act with respect to their information? There are some clear areas of care in which consideration of breaches of confidence might be made, for instance, in tracing the contacts of people likely to have been exposed to the same infectious agents as a patient. Examples of contact tracing include identifying sexual partners of individuals newly diagnosed with life-threatening sexually transmitted infections, such as human immunodeficiency virus, and the tracing of all contacts, intimate and casual, of individuals with diseases such as tuberculosis.

Variations on the exercise of the right to confidentiality tell us something about the weight we might apply to consideration of individuality when these considerations come up against considerations of the wider public good, as Dworkin (1987) suggests.

....

Case study: when breaking a confidence is in the public interest

Beauchamp and Childress (2012) report on the tragic case of Tatiana Tarasoff, whose death gives us good cause to consider the scope of the right to confidentiality. Tatiana was a student at Berkeley University, California, and had kissed a fellow student, Prosenjit Poddar, during New Year celebrations. Poddar interpreted this as meaning they were in a relationship and was distraught to find Tatiana did not think the same way. Poddar started neglecting himself and showing signs of mental distress. He was convinced to start seeing a university psychologist, Dr Lawrence Moore. Poddar told Dr Moore that he planned to kill Tatiana during one session and Dr Moore informed the police. The police questioned Poddar, who told police he had changed his mind and he was released on the promise he did not go anywhere near Tatiana.

Moore's boss, Dr Powelson, instructed the university medical team not to try to have Poddar detained and Poddar stopped seeing Dr Moore. In October 1969 Poddar went to Tatiana's house and stabbed her to death.

....

This very sad case points to another reason we are not obliged to maintain patient confidences at all costs. In the case of Tatiana Tarasoff, the clear message which emerged was not that of detaining Poddar, but that Tatiana had not been made aware of the threat on her life because of issues relating to professional–client confidentiality.

The example of the death of Tatiana Tarasoff gives us pause for thought. What are the competing rights in play here and how might we choose between them? While Poddar has a clear right to privacy and to having his confidences maintained, there are important competing rights at play here too. The psychologist has the right (or perhaps duty) to break this confidence in order to protect some wider public good and Tatiana certainly had the right to know that threats were being made against her life. Her right to self-preservation certainly seems to be somewhat more important than any right Poddar might lay claim to.

Chapter summary

This chapter has demonstrated the existence of rights in the care setting and has explored one explanation, interest theories, as to the origins of these rights. We have seen how rights take different forms and therefore place different obligations on the nurse and other providers of care. We have seen how rights operate primarily to protect the individual from interference by others which is neither justifiable nor wanted.

This chapter has further demonstrated that rights cannot be evoked in an arbitrary manner. Rather, rights should be applied considering their scope, importance and impact on the individual claiming the right and those affected by it. We have also seen that at least one ethical basis for rights, interests, may continue to be in force even after the person holding the interest has stopped being aware of their existence.

Activities: brief outline answers

Activity 5.1 Reflection

This may seem like an odd question and one with no real answer, except that it does have an answer. Today you are reading this book and this suggests you are free to do so. This in turn suggests you have a right to choose what you read; this is a form of the right to freedom of expression. You may have been out and about today and experienced no interference from other people; this is because you are at liberty to go about your business unimpeded and being at liberty to do so is an expression of your right to live your life without undue interference.

Activity 5.2 Critical thinking

This is a hard issue to grapple with. On the basis of legal and special rights, people who do not have citizenship do not have any right to claim healthcare provision. On a more human level, it is clear that all people have a right to health. What this right will amount to in reality will depend very much on where the person lives and the availability of resources. It is hard as a nurse who is tuned in to meeting need whenever and wherever it arises to see beyond this to the impact of a free healthcare for everyone system.

Activity 5.5 Decision making

This scenario demonstrates the tension between the technical and the contextual decision making that forms some of the dilemmas seen in nursing. It is obvious that Gordon's physical best interests would be best served by an increase in help but that, in context, as a private and independent couple Gordon and Nicola would not welcome the intrusion. They regard their independence as reflective of who they are as people and do not want to be seen as *people who need help* – this is an interest of theirs. The answer here for the student nurse is obvious: this is a discussion which needs to be had with a trained member of staff. There are issues such as Gordon's safety at stake here; there is also a need to ensure that Gordon and Nicola understand the nature of the help available and that they are making an informed choice. If the choice is genuine then it is a decision they have to be allowed to make. If you are concerned about Gordon's and Nicola's competence there would be good reason to involve a mental health professional in the assessment.

Activity 5.6 Decision making

This is a tricky scenario as there is no evidence of neglect, just some difficulties with Gordon getting the care he needs. On the one hand, it is in his experiential best interests to be somewhere safer and, on the other, it may be in his critical best interests to stay with Nicola. However, as Dresser (2010) points out, he may no longer care about the critical best interest. That said, it is always possible that someone's critical best interests outlive their capacity to experience or care about them – that is to say they remain in force to protect the integrity (congruence) of the way the person wanted to lead their life.

Further reading

Buka, P (2008) *Patients' Rights, Law and Ethics for Nurses: A Practical Guide.* Florida: CRC Press. An informative look at the law and rights.

Griffith, R and Tengnah, C (2014) *Law and Professional Issues in Nursing*, 3rd edn. Transforming Nursing Practice Series. London: Sage.

Useful websites

www.liberty-human-rights.org.uk/human-rights/what-are-human-rights/international-human-rights
There is some background to human rights here as well as links to the European Declaration on Human Rights.

www.gov.uk/government/publications/the-nhs-constitution-for-england
Visit this site to review the NHS Constitution.

www.un.org/en/documents/udhr
The United Nations Universal Declaration of Human Rights.

Chapter 6
Key areas in healthcare ethics (protecting and promoting autonomy)

Peter Ellis

NMC Standards for Pre-registration Nursing Education

This chapter will address the following competencies:

Domain 1: Generic standards for competence
3. All nurses must support and promote the health, wellbeing, rights and dignity of people, groups, communities and populations. These include people whose lives are affected by ill health, disability, ageing, death and dying. Nurses must understand how these activities influence public health.
4. All nurses must work in partnership with service users, carers, families, groups, communities and organisations. They must manage risk and promote health and wellbeing while aiming to empower choices that promote self-care and safety.

Domain 2: Communication and interpersonal skills
1. All nurses must build partnerships and therapeutic relationships through safe, effective and non-discriminatory communication. They must take account of individual differences, capabilities and needs.
4. All nurses must recognise when people are anxious or in distress and respond effectively, using therapeutic principles, to promote their wellbeing, manage personal safety and resolve conflict. They must use effective communication strategies and negotiation techniques to achieve best outcomes, respecting the dignity and human rights of all concerned. They must know when to consult a third party and how to make referrals for advocacy, mediation or arbitration.

Domain 3: Nursing practice and decision making
9. All nurses must be able to recognise when a person is at risk and in need of extra support and protection and take reasonable steps to protect them from abuse.

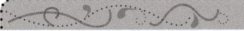

NMC Essential Skills Clusters

This chapter will address the following ESCs:

Care, compassion and communication
Patients/clients can trust a newly registered graduate nurse to:
2. Engage them as partners in care. Should they be unable to meet their own needs then the nurse will ensure that these are addressed in accordance with the known wishes of the patient/client or in their best interests.
6. Listen, and provide information that is clear, accurate and meaningful at a level at which the patient/client can understand.
8. Ensure that their consent will be sought prior to care or treatment being given and that their rights will be respected.

Chapter aims

After reading this chapter you will be able to:

*   discuss why autonomy is such an important concept;
*   identify the barriers which arise in practice preventing people from the exercise of autonomy;
*   consider situations in practice which require you to promote or protect the autonomy of others;
*   begin to understand the role of the student nurse, or nurse, in empowering, advocating for or gaining consent from patients.

Introduction

We have established in this book that ethics is a live issue. Ethics is both a response to and a requirement of living in societies. We have further explored issues around the importance of the individual nurse as an **agent** of ethics, as well as an agent in general. By agent we mean someone who is free and capable of making decisions for and about him/herself. We have also seen, in the previous chapter, how rights might operate to protect some important aspects of being human. In this chapter we explore how nurses can protect and promote **agency** in the people they come into contact with.

In this chapter we will explore four of the cornerstones of ethical activity which contribute to agency within the healthcare setting: autonomy, empowerment, advocacy and consent. These cornerstones derive from, and demonstrate the supremacy of, the *individual*. This westernised view of **personhood** states that individuals are at liberty to live their own lives as they see fit and, in so far as they are able, to make decisions about how they live their life and what is done by, for and to them.

Some ethicists would call this a libertarian view of ethics; that is to say, it is concerned with a view of ethics which sees the liberty of individuals to live their lives as they see fit is more important than most – if not all – other ethical and legal obligations.

The themes of empowerment, advocacy and consent are all connected by notions which relate to the principle of autonomy and therefore this is where we will start.

Autonomy

The word autonomy comes from the Greek words *auto* and *nomos*, which mean *self-rule* (or *self-law*); in the literal sense, autonomy means the ability to make decisions about oneself and to act upon these decisions.

Autonomy is something which for a large part we take for granted. Every day we make many decisions about many things for and about ourselves. We decide when to get up and what to wear, whether to shower or bath, what we will have for breakfast, and so on. Of course these decisions have some constraints upon them: when we get out of bed may be dictated by the fact that we have to be somewhere, perhaps at work or university; what we wear will depend on where we are going and the weather; the choice of bath or shower might be determined by availability and time; while what we eat will depend to a large extent on what we have in the cupboard. This does not mean we are not autonomous – it just means autonomy has some practical boundaries.

Some philosophers who subscribe to a view of human activity called **determinism** think people only act in ways which are *determined* by things which have gone before (we are products of our past and have no **free will**). Whether this is true does not matter to the nurse since the exercise of autonomy by patients, whether they have free will or they are deterministic, relates to who these people are (it is coherent to them). Our code and our values exhort us to protect the exercise of autonomy, however and whenever it is exercised, so long as the patient exercising it has capacity (see later).

Respecting the autonomy of others and their freedom to make choices about what they do and when would seem to be a reasonable requirement of the nursing profession. After all, the first line of *The Code: Professional Standards of Practice and Behaviour for Nurses and Midwives* (NMC, 2015) states nurses must *treat people as individuals and respect their dignity*.

What the Nursing and Midwifery Council (NMC) is meaning by *respect their dignity* is little more than allowing people to make choices about their care – that is, allowing them the dignity of choice. Treating *people as individuals* means these choices should be made by each person singularly and with reference to what each person wants and not in response to what we, as nurses, want. Allowing people to make choices about their care requires that healthcare professionals provide environments of care in which autonomy is actively promoted. This notion of autonomy sits well with modern nursing rhetoric and practices regarding patient-centred care which is more than merely allowing choice, it is about actively engaging people to ensure they make the choice they want about their care for their own reasons.

....

Case study: respecting autonomy

Winifred is on placement in a home which provides care to residents who have varying degrees of learning difficulty. Winifred is asked by Jo, the lead carer, to help one of the residents, Cynthia, dress. Winifred goes to Cynthia's room, rummages through the drawers and wardrobe and selects an outfit. Cynthia starts crying and shouting and is obviously very cross when Winifred starts to dress her. Jo comes in to see what all the fuss is about. She asks Winifred why she is dressing Cynthia in those particular clothes. Winifred responds 'because they look nice'. Jo suggests to Winifred that she might like to let Cynthia choose her own clothes.

....

Activity 6.1	*Reflection*

Taking the case study as a guide, put yourself in Winifred's position. Consider what she has done and why Cynthia might have responded in the way that she did. Now reflect on not only what Winifred did, but also the motivations behind her action and consider how she (or you) might better approach this sort of situation in the future and what motivations might underpin this.

There are some possible answers to all activities at the end of the chapter, unless otherwise indicated.

What this scenario shows is the need to consider not only that people might be able to exercise autonomy even when we think they might not, but also that in promoting that autonomy we, as nurses, are doing what is right by them. This is especially important in the care setting where, by virtue of illness and the nature of care environments, the opportunity to exercise autonomy is more often than not significantly reduced. Not only is this good ethically, but promoting autonomy can also be good for many people in helping them overcome or adapt to disease and ill health.

A further, and very important, reason why autonomy is important is the fact that respecting people's autonomy is one way in which we can demonstrate what many ethicists call **respect for persons**. Respect for persons implies that, through respecting the right of individuals to make choices, we are respecting them as human beings. There are a great many arguments as to why we owe other people ethical consideration, some of which we discussed in Chapter 1.

Respect for autonomy is therefore not about respect for a principle or concept; it is good for many people in terms of recovery or adaptation to ill health and it is a tangible way in which we as nurses can demonstrate our respect for people. Autonomy is not, however, the same as freedom. Freedom is being in a position to be able to act as one wishes, while autonomy is seen by some philosophers as referring to something more globally about the person (Dworkin, 1988) – independence, the ability to choose and subsequently to act upon the choices made.

This latter definition of autonomy then creates a triumvirate of possible points of intervention for the nurse: promoting independence (perhaps by encouraging and supporting); allowing choice (by providing more than one option); and enabling action (either by not interfering or by providing physical or emotional support). These constituent elements which contribute to the protection, promotion and enactment of autonomy can be seen in action when nurses choose to empower, advocate for or gain consent from patients.

Empowerment

Empowerment is a term widely used in health and social care to identify activities in which caring professionals prompt and support those in their care to take control of what is happening to them. Empowerment literally means to give power to. Practically speaking, in the care setting empowerment is probably best thought of as the action which occurs when patients or clients are encouraged to discuss their own preferences for care once they are in full receipt of the facts about the treatment options available to them. It may also be thought of as enabling patients to engage in activities which support the choices they have made.

Important examples of empowerment in the physical sense, as hinted at above, might include referral to other professionals and agencies who can provide strategies or physical tools which support patients to enact their personal choices. Instances of empowering referrals might include: to the physiotherapist who provides a walking frame which *empowers* the patient to take control of walking, or to the social worker who provides home care which allows the patient to leave the hospital.

Empowerment then has a physical as well as psychological dimension. This dichotomy of meaning sits well with standard 4 of Domain 1, generic standards for competence, cited at the start of the chapter, which exhorts nurses both to *work in partnership with* and *empower choices that promote self-care and safety* (NMC, 2010).

Many discussions of empowerment also include discussions about advocacy, with some commentators seeing very little difference between the two. Empowerment differs from advocacy in one important way: in advocacy (as we shall see) someone represents the patient's view to others, whereas in empowerment patients are encouraged to present their views for themselves.

> ### Scenario: empowering the patient
>
> *Dorothy is an 80-year-old woman who has been admitted to the ear, nose and throat ward with recurrent nasal bleeds. Edith is sitting with Dorothy when the registrar visits her to discuss her treatment options. When the registrar has finished, he asks Dorothy what she would like to do. Dorothy turns to Edith and asks: 'What would you do?'*
>
> *Edith asks Dorothy if she has understood what has been told to her. She says 'not really'. Edith suggests the registrar returns to talk to Dorothy later once Edith has had had the opportunity to explain her options to her. Dorothy is a little worried by this turn of events and asks Edith to decide what she should do; Edith is clear in her mind that Dorothy should decide on her course of action herself and spends some time explaining the options to her.*

> Consider the preceding scenario. Why might it not be reasonable for Edith to make the decision on behalf of Dorothy? What is it Edith is trying to achieve? If Edith were to make the decision for Dorothy, would she be demonstrating a lack of respect for her as a person?

Sometimes the easy thing to do is to make decisions for the other person and sometimes this is the *right* thing to do. In the scenario described above, Edith could have decided to make Dorothy's decision for her, but doing so would mean that she failed to promote Dorothy's independence and autonomy and therefore this *may* not be the *right* thing to do.

This scenario makes two key points about empowerment. First, it encourages people to speak for themselves and second, to empower individuals they must not only be given information, but they must also understand it. There is a saying that *knowledge is power* and in sharing knowledge as nurses we can em*power* our patients to make decisions which affect their lives.

As a student nurse, you may feel you have little to offer to your patients in the way of empowering them. You may feel you have little power yourself and therefore it is not something you can become involved in. This overlooks a number of important points about the nature of the relationship between nurses and patients in the care setting as well as the nature and meaning of empowerment.

The first issue is quite conceptual, but is very important. Empowerment should not be seen by nurses as us giving something to someone else; rather it should be seen as a way of ensuring people exercise that which is rightly already theirs. Environments of care often rob people of the ability to exercise their autonomy – disempower them – because of the way in which they are set up. What is required, according to Christensen and Hewitt-Taylor (2006), is for individuals (care professionals) and organisations to alter their beliefs and behaviours. A good example of this is the **sick role** which people adopt on entering the hospital setting but which in many cases is not necessary.

Concept summary: the sick role

Talcott Parsons (1951), a **functionalist** sociologist, coined the term the *sick role*. In Parsons' view, once we are sick we are allowed to withdraw from our usual responsibilities within society, but we also have a corresponding obligation to find a way to make ourselves better. In tandem with the obligation to get well again, we are also obliged to allow those who have the expertise (i.e. doctors) to make decisions about what is best for us in order to achieve this.

While this concept may grate with many of us, it is a good observation of how the behaviour of even highly motivated and competent people can change when they are ill. Consider the patient who walks on to the ward, changes into pyjamas and is then incapable of walking to the X-ray department!

Second, by empowering people what we often mean is merely sharing information with them, or ensuring that others share information with them. This information is often only about rephrasing things patients have already been told into language they understand and reminding them that they have choices (more on this in the section on consent, below).

The final point we want to make is about the nature of the caring relationship. The sole purpose of nursing is to provide care for individuals so they can achieve their full potential. This is not always about physical potential, but psychological as well as spiritual. Empowerment in this sense is about enabling the whole person.

Case study: the empowered older person

Bernard Jordan, an 89-year-old veteran of the Second World War, had been unable to arrange to return to France for the D-Day 70th-anniversary commemorations in 2014. Instead of just watching on the television, he decided to walk out of his care home and made his own way to Portsmouth where he found and joined a group of fellow veterans returning to Normandy (Sawyer, 2014).

This real-life story sends an important message to nurses – that we should never underestimate the need to exercise autonomy nor who in our care is empowered.

Advocacy

Whether nurses should act as **advocates** is controversial in some quarters of nursing. Some commentators suggest that nurses must always act as the patient's advocate, others that it is not the nurse's role to act as advocate, some that advocacy is in itself disempowering of patients (Allmark and Klarzynski, 1992), while many nurses believe it is one of many roles which nurse *have* to fulfil.

The NMC is, however, unequivocal about this, stating within *The Code* (NMC, 2015) that nurses must act as advocates for the vulnerable, challenging poor practice and discriminatory attitudes and behaviour relating to their care.

So what does it mean to be an advocate? When we act as advocates we represent the interests of another person as if they were our own. This requires putting to one side any ideas, feelings, thoughts and beliefs we might have and acting purely as someone else's mouthpiece. One of the challenges which faces the nurse advocate is having to represent a view to which we are totally opposed (Schwartz, 2002).

Activity 6.3   *Critical thinking*

Bearing in mind what we have said about what it means to advocate, what do you think are some of the problems facing nurses thinking about being advocates for their patients? Consider here not only the issues of understanding the other point of view, but what a nurse needs to do to be an advocate in situations where there is some disagreement as to what is the right course of action in a particular situation. You may be able to recall a situation like this from your own practice experience.

The tensions for the nurse acting as the patient's mouthpiece are varied and real. They can arise out of the disagreement between the patient and the nurse and between the patient and the healthcare team in general. The important issue to consider for the nurse, or nursing student, is that it is the *act of advocacy* which our code of conduct requires of us; *The Code* (NMC, 2015) does not tell us the detail of *what* we should advocate.

Scenario: everyday advocacy in nursing

Gareth is a student nurse who is working on an elective surgery orthopaedic ward. Various patients have been to theatre in the morning and have returned to the ward. On return to the ward one patient, Giles, says he is in considerable pain and wants some painkillers. Gareth approaches his mentor Wendy and asks if Giles can have some pain relief. After reviewing Giles's chart, Wendy says 'no, he is not due any more for 2 hours'. Gareth is a little surprised and returns to Giles to tell him, but on approaching the bed it is clear Giles is still in pain. Gareth goes back to Wendy and tells her Giles is still in pain and that they should get him some other form of analgesia written up. Wendy relents and pages the doctor.

This is a simple and frequent scenario which demonstrates advocacy is not always something complex or controversial. In this scenario Gareth recognises that Giles is in pain and wants some pain relief; he advocates for Giles to his mentor and is subsequently persistent when his initial approach is turned down. In this case Gareth is acting in accordance with *The Code* (NMC, 2015), which suggests what we should 'act in partnership with those receiving care, helping them to access relevant health and social care, information and support when they need it'.

Concept summary: reasons for advocacy

- Patient is vulnerable.
- Patient lacks ability to communicate clearly.
- Advocate may be in meetings where the patient is not.
- Patient may not understand medical terminology.
- Patient is frightened.
- Patient may choose not to represent themselves.

One of the key criticisms of advocacy lies in the fact that we take on the mantle of representing the patient and as a result patients do not represent themselves. This suggests that we as nurses take the power from patients and, instead of *empowering* them to represent themselves, we infantilise them by acting in a manner which some regard as **parentalistic**.

Advocacy and empowerment could be thought of as being on a continuum which recognises the supremacy of patients in any decision making which is about them. This interpretation of advocacy and empowerment recognises the central importance of personal autonomy, and *respect for persons*, and is in essence a practical one. This observation recognises that people need both autonomy and understanding in order to inform their choice. That the choices people make are heard and acted upon is perhaps, in the great scheme of things, more important than exactly how these choices are given voice.

Consent

Consent is a fundamental aspect of everything we do as nurses, from the taking of a temperature to administration of medication and dressing of wounds. In fact, as UK law stands, just touching patients without their consent is battery (Avery, 2013). *The Code* (NMC, 2015) also reminds us to: *make sure that you get properly informed consent and document it before carrying out any action.*

In this section of the chapter we will explore not only what consent is, but also the multiple facets which go into gaining consent. For the most part this discussion relates to adults; however, many of the principles apply equally well to children.

The word *consent* comes from the Latin word *consentire*, which means 'feeling together'. This togetherness comes about as a result of a choice which is made whereby both parties in an arrangement agree to something happening.

The right to *autonomy*/principle of *respect of persons* is bound up with *informed consent* (Eby, 2000) and therefore the gaining of consent is not only a legal requirement, it is a means of demonstrating ethical activity on our part. In many ways, gaining consent is the ultimate expression of respect, not only for autonomy and persons but also the principles which underpin advocacy and empowerment, as previously discussed.

Consent is not simply the act of getting someone to agree to something; in fact, one might argue that it is quite the opposite. The gaining of consent should take place in an atmosphere of choice, mutual trust and understanding and therefore 'getting someone to agree' should not enter the equation. Consent is therefore by definition a multifaceted process; each of its elements must be in place in order for the consent to be truly valid.

The gaining of consent should not be considered as a one-off activity. People have the right to change their mind and also to withdraw from prior agreements; in this respect consent is a complex and dynamic process which nurses should not take for granted. As well as being complex, consent may take a number of different forms and the practising nurse will need to be sensitive to these.

Implicit and explicit consent

When thinking about consent, most people think about the formal process undertaken prior to a surgical or invasive medical procedure. This process follows a set of guidelines in a particular order in order to obtain a signature which is used to demonstrate individuals have agreed to something happening to them. As alluded to at the start of this section, everything we do as nurses requires the permission of the patient, but not everything requires consent to be as explicit as that gained prior to surgery.

Activity 6.4   *Reflection*

Consider some of the day-to-day activities you have engaged in today. How many of them contain an element of consent or cooperation? How is that consent demonstrated? Consider the same issues in the practice setting and when working as a healthcare professional: how do you ensure that when you do something to or with patients it is something to which they have agreed?

Human interaction is peppered with examples of implicit consent, e.g. sitting in the dentist chair and opening our mouth. Mutual consent and mutual cooperation are two of the backbones of a well-functioning society. Being receptive to signs of consent is a fundamental aspect of good nursing communication, as is detecting when an individual is not happy with what is happening to him or her!

Elements of consent

In order to be sure that consent is valid and the people we are caring for are exercising their autonomy in allowing us to work with them, it is important for nurses to establish that a number of criteria are met. The criteria which indicate consent is indeed genuine take into account the ability of the person to make choices, the influences affecting how the individual chooses and the need for there to be a choice to be made.

Where any of the elements of consent are missing it is questionable as to whether true consent has been gained. In some instances the role of the nurse is to gain patient consent and in others it is to ensure that consent has been gained properly and that it is genuine.

Concept summary: the elements of consent

- Capacity;
- Information;
- Understanding;
- Freedom from coercion;
- Freedom of choice.

The concept summary above identifies five criteria which need to be met for consent to be valid (note: other commentators identify different criteria). The rest of the chapter is devoted to exploring each of these elements.

Capacity

The first requirement for there to be consent is that the person giving it has the capacity to do so. In this sense capacity does not mean time, it means mental ability. Capacity is sometimes referred to as agency, where agency means the ability of a person to exercise choice. In this context the person is seen as an agent, someone who acts out the choices s/he has made.

In the healthcare setting the ability to make health-related decisions may be one step removed from agency in that individual patients will require the input of care professionals in order to realise whatever choice it is they have made. In this respect capacity in the healthcare setting is sometimes referred to as **decisional capacity**.

The Mental Capacity Act 2005, in force in England and Wales, provides a good guide to what is expected from all professionals with respect to establishing the capacity of an individual.

Concept summary: the Mental Capacity Act 2005

The five principles from section 1 of the Mental Capacity Act 2005 state:

1. A person must be assumed to have capacity unless it is established that he/she lacks capacity.
2. A person is not to be treated as unable to make a decision unless all practicable steps to help him/her to do so have been taken without success.
3. A person is not to be treated as unable to make a decision merely because he/she makes an unwise decision.
4. An act done, or decision made, under this Act for or on behalf of a person who lacks capacity must be done, or made, in his/her best interests.
5. Before the act is done, or the decision is made, regard must be had to whether the purpose for which it is needed can be as effectively achieved in a way that is less restrictive of the person's rights and freedom of action.

Scenario: questioning capacity

Mario lives in an assisted-living setting with two other men with learning disability. Mario has struck up a friendship with some young men at the local pub and is frequently seen there buying them drinks. Mario does appear to be buying his friends more drinks than they buy him in return. This gets back to Mario's assisted-living support worker, Charlene, who is concerned that Mario is being exploited. When Charlene raises the issue, Mario is adamant that he knows what he is doing, the money is his to spend as he sees fit and anyway his young friends do not have as much money as he does.

Usually it is obvious that someone has, or does not have, capacity. There are, however, many grey areas which involve issues such as mental illness, learning disability, age and levels of consciousness in which it is difficult to know whether the person is competent or not – or indeed if they lack capacity only temporarily. In Mario's case he makes a coherent argument as to why he should be left to do as he sees fit which might, assuming there are no other reasons to doubt his capacity, suggest he is merely exercising his free will.

While it is beyond the scope of this book to explore each eventuality, it is important you understand there is no blanket answer to whether mental illness, learning disability, age and levels of consciousness lead to incapacity. Invariably the difficult cases need to be assessed on their own merits, as in Mario's case, and, as the Mental Capacity Act 2005 points out, just because someone makes what we might consider to be a bad choice does not mean that s/he lacks capacity!

Information

Information giving is a fundamental part of the role of the nurse. Information can come in many forms and withholding information from individuals is under most circumstances the wrong thing to do. When considering consent it is not just the type and nature of the information that is given which are important; scope also plays a large role in supporting the ability of the individual to exercise choice. What does this mean?

If choice is part of the consent process then people must be presented with the information they need to make a choice. This will mean not only providing information about the treatment or intervention we usually give, but also any other options the individual might choose (within reason). As well as the alternatives with their attendant outcomes, choice requires us to remind patients that they do not have to have any treatments/interventions at all if they do not wish to.

If we consider the ethical principle of *respect for persons*, which we identified as being the principle which gives rise to *respect for autonomy*, then withholding information which an individual might use in the process of making a decision could demonstrate a lack of respect both for the *person* and for his or her *autonomy*.

There is great emphasis these days in healthcare settings on providing information in different formats or in providing interpreters. This is not merely about getting information across for the sake of getting information across, it is also about ensuring people have access to the information they need to make choices and exercise consent.

Understanding

While the giving of information is an important part of the role of the nurse, making sure that the information given is understood is absolutely fundamental to ethical nursing practice. If you recall the scenario involving Dorothy, at the start of this chapter, the ethical issue which presented itself to Edith was not entirely about empowering or advocating for Dorothy, but more about the fact that Dorothy had not understood what had been said to her by the doctor.

Without understanding there is little chance for patients to make choices which reflect what they really want from a situation.

Scenario: information and understanding

Mervin is being consented to have a contract enhanced magnetic resonance imaging (MRI) scan for recurrent headaches. Jo, a student nurse, sits in while the doctor 'gains consent'. When the paperwork is done and the doctor has gone Mervin asks Jo what 'tumour and contrast enhanced MRI' mean. It is clear to Jo that while Mervin has been given the information he needs to make a decisions about the operation, he has not understood it. She asks her mentor to speak to the doctor so that Mervin can be consented properly.

The preceding scenario demonstrates how information and understanding are not the same. Ethically, in order to demonstrate respect for persons, all care professionals are obliged to ensure any information they give to a patient is understood. Understanding for consent goes beyond an understanding of the medical/nursing processes on offer; it extends to ensuring that patients understand they have choices and the freedom to exercise those choices.

Freedom from coercion

While it is probably true to say that purposeful, explicit coercion is rare in the practice setting, inadvertent and implicit coercion clearly is not. Earlier in the chapter we discussed some of the influences on the individual in the care setting which arise out of the cultures of care. These *care-specific* influences occur in tandem with societal norms of behaviour to exert a very real influence on the ways in which people behave.

A dictionary definition of coercion would include notions of forcing someone to act in a certain way as a result of a threat or some other pressure being brought to bear. In the rest of this section we will examine the nature of some of these pressures and what they might mean for the consent process.

Scenario: the impact of coercion on decision making

Frank is an 84-year-old widower who lives alone. Frank has had hypertension for years and as a result has developed chronic kidney disease. Frank is approaching the point at which he will need to have dialysis to stay alive, although he also knows he has the choice not to be treated and have symptom management if he wishes. Frank has discussed his options with the nurses in the advanced kidney care clinic and has opted to have conservative (symptom control) management of his kidney disease.

Frank's family are not happy with his decision and tell him so, especially his granddaughter who is quite vocal and tells the nursing team that they are killing her granddad. As a result of pressure from his family Frank changes his mind and goes on to haemodialysis. This makes him very tired and miserable.

Situations such as Frank's are very common in the care setting where people are understandably upset about the fact that a loved one may be dying. We see two issues influencing the ultimate decision Frank makes: the first is what he wants for himself and the second is how he tries to please his family.

Activity 6.5   *Critical thinking*

Having identified what coercion is and some of the forms it takes, consider the scenario featuring Frank and his eventual decision to undergo dialysis in order to appease his family. Does this appear to you to be a case of coercion? Is it right that Frank's decision should be influenced by his family? Is there a middle ground which might be attained here?

But what exactly constitutes coercion in healthcare practice? The answer to this lies both within the context of the situation and also the people involved. Coercion is a function of many different factors but when boiled down to its barest essentials coercion usually arises out of the exercise of power.

Power comes in many different forms and may influence people in very many different ways. The relationship between the care professional and the patient is not evenly balanced, with patients choosing to do what the nurse asks in order to please him or her. Simple examples might include responding to the ward nurse who says 'put out your arm so I can do your blood pressure' or when a clinic nurse recruits patients from her clinic to be involved in her MSc study. In terms of taking the blood pressure, this is probably in the best interests of the patient, but the manner of the approach suggests little room for manoeuvre. In the second instance, participating in the study may not be to the benefit of patients, but they feel they cannot refuse as they are in a dependent relationship with the nurse.

We saw in Chapter 1 how professional identity can lead to people creating personas which are binary; that is identities which identify other people who are not like us as other. One example of this 'other' is the grateful patient who accepts the care we offer because we are the professional and they are not. The dangers of accepting this as a reasonable way to operate are all too evident in the healthcare setting.

Neither of the previous examples demonstrates anything particularly unethical per se (although the clinic nurse would have had to gain ethical approval for her study), but what they do is highlight how easy it is for coercion to slide into everyday practice without the nurse being aware. Perhaps more tangible examples of coercion include situations in which money is promised.

Case studies: coercion in action?

In 2006 a number of healthy volunteers were recruited to be guinea pigs in a trial which involved the first human injections of a newly developed monoclonal antibody agent called TGN1412. Participation in the trial was rewarded with a fee of £2,000 (Emanuel and Miller, 2007).

(continued)

---

continued . . .

> A cursory search on the internet using the terms 'kidneys for sale' identifies a number of stories of people from around the world, including the UK, who are actively trying to sell one of their kidneys for cash. One website offers $70,000–80,000 and the chance to 'pay all your debts'.

What the two examples above demonstrate is the potential for coercion arising out of the offer of money. While it may be fair to raise counter-arguments about people receiving just reward for a service rendered, the relative poverty of the people who take up offers of money to do things – which under ordinary circumstances they would not choose to do if not paid – does give cause for some ethical discomfort.

Coercion in the consent process is usually a lot more subtle and may arise out of the failure to provide sufficient information about alternatives and the right to exercise choice. The coercion here arises out of the implicit assumption that what we as nurses are offering is what the patient *should* do.

So avoiding coercion in the consent process is quite a lot more complex than just not threatening patients. It involves some considerable thought from nurses about how they exercise both power and provide information. As we saw in the activity featuring Frank, one of the ways in which the nurse can enable the patient is to enable the family as well. Patients are entitled to, and do, consult their friends and family when important decisions need to be made – information for loved ones is one tool which will allow them to become part of a constructive decision-making process which is less likely to involve coercion resulting from a lack of understanding of the real issues.

Note: not all coercion in the care setting is bad, with some coercion, e.g. providing sweets as an incentive for a child to sit still whilst being vaccinated, being done with the patient's best interests at heart. Nevertheless, implicit and unconscious acts of coercion are commonplace in nursing practice and are at odds both with notions of patient-centred care and respect for persons. For example, it is easy to say to a patient 'I would do so and so' or 'it would be easier if you did …'; although these actions are not in themselves unethical, in the context of the power difference at work in the care setting they can prove coercive.

Activity 6.6   *Reflection*

Reflect upon the examples given here and think about your own practice. Do you always ask rather than tell? Do you coerce patients into doing things to make your life easier? Do you always ensure patients understand what you tell them?

Since the answers to this activity are personal to you, there is no specimen answer at the end of the chapter.

Freedom of choice

To have the freedom to choose, there has to be more than one option available to an individual. In many cases this will mean having the recommended treatment or not. Freedom to choose suggests that the options open to the individual are equally weighted and that the decision is one of preference, rather than necessity.

In reality this is often not the case where care is involved. Sometimes this is because of the nature of the problem the person presents with and sometimes it is because the system only allows limited choice. As Lynch (2011, p. 38) points out, *'Patient choice' means that the patient may choose from the range of options offered to them. It does not mean that the patient can demand a particular course of treatment.* Although of course any patient who has capacity may choose to be left alone.

> ### Scenario: providing reasonable choices
>
> *Gunther is almost 90 years old. He is admitted to the orthopaedic ward after a fall at home which resulted in him having a fractured neck of femur. The orthopaedic surgeons tell Gunther that, given the location and nature of the fracture, the rational option for him is to have a total hip replacement after which he will be up and walking in days. The alternative is to pin and plate the fracture, which is likely to have a similar result, but which might not last as long and given Gunther's age might break in any subsequent fall.*
>
> *Gunther refuses both options as he wants to be put in traction and the fracture allowed to heal naturally, as he had seen happen to his brother Sven when they were boys. The surgeons explain that at his age prolonged bed rest will probably result in him dying from pneumonia and that this is not an option.*

This scenario makes the important point that, while patients are free to make choices about their health, there does need to be some rational empirical evidence as to what these choices might reasonably be in many cases. Gunther may of course choose to follow his initial choice, as he has capacity, but he will have to take the attendant risk.

The flip-side scenario is one where the healthcare professionals fail to tell patients about their choices, or fail to provide sufficient information about a procedure to allow them to exercise freedom of choice.

Activity 6.7   *Communication*

> Simon is a junior doctor on a urology ward. He is asked to gain written informed consent from Daniel for a transurethral resection of prostate (TURP), which he does. Daniel is prepared for theatre and the porter arrives. Ben, a student nurse, asks Daniel if he has signed a consent form and whether he understands the potential side effects and complications arising from a TURP. He also asks if alternative treatment strategies were discussed. Daniel says he signed the consent, but did not understand that there might be alternatives nor indeed that there are side effects from a TURP. What should Ben do?

In this scenario, it is not only the lack of information which limits Daniel's freedom; it is the nature of the interaction which has robbed him of any say in what he does. Freedom to choose in this case is not just about saying yes or no; it is also about being in the position where it is clear that the professional is interested in allowing patients to exercise that choice of their own free will. Yet again this brings us back to considering how allowing a person to exercise free choice is one way of demonstrating respect for autonomy.

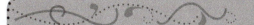

Chapter summary

This chapter has explored the interrelated topics of autonomy, empowerment, advocacy and consent. Throughout the chapter we have seen the common thread, which has been the exercise of autonomy. We have seen that respect for autonomy, and for persons, underpins each of the other activities discussed here.

We have seen there are areas of concern in terms of the philosophy and ethics of each of these topic areas and that not all ethical theorists and nurses agree with either the concepts or exercise of all of these topic areas.

What is clear from the discussion is that what we do as nurses for and with our patients requires us to communicate with them at a level they can understand. Failure to do this demonstrates a lack of respect and is contrary to the ethical practice of nursing.

Autonomy is a live issue in healthcare provision. Some readers will see this as arising directly out of imbalances of power within the nurse–patient relationship and perhaps even as a result of blatant abuse. While in some instances this has proven to be true, we should end the chapter remembering how complex care is and how rapidly care practices change. The complexity and ever-changing nature of care on their own are, however, enough of a reason why nurses should engage with practices which both promote and protect the autonomy of patients. As we have seen, much of the requirement which goes towards championing autonomy is related to giving information and checking understanding. It is unlikely, therefore, that this important role of the nurse will ever come to an end.

Activities: brief outline answers

Activity 6.1 Reflection

In the scenario Winifred makes the assumption that Cynthia is incapable of making decisions about what to wear. She further assumes that the best thing to do therefore is make those choices for her in order that she can, as she has been asked to do, get Cynthia dressed. While she may have been acting from kindly motives, she has failed to promote or respect Cynthia's autonomy. Winifred might have asked Cynthia what she would like to wear; she might have suggested some clothes and waited for a positive response before just going ahead and attempting to dress her, as if she were merely a doll.

Activity 6.2 Critical thinking

While it is not wrong to help patients make a decision about their care or treatment, it is important that patients make the choice for us to help them as a conscious decision and not just because they are uncertain about what is happening. In this case Dorothy is not able to exercise her autonomy because she does not understand what is being said to her, not because she is incapable of doing so. Edith is trying to empower Dorothy by making sure she has options; it may prove that Dorothy chooses to exercise the option of letting Edith decide on her care once she has understood the options. Under these circumstances she would still be exercising her autonomy.

Activity 6.3 Critical thinking

When a nurse decides to act as an advocate for a patient there are a large number of tensions which can arise. These may be because the nurse does not agree with what the patient is asking him or her to advocate (that is, s/he thinks the patient is making the wrong decision); the nurse may agree with what the patient wants but the rest of the healthcare team may not and so this requires the nurse to stand the patient's ground against his or her colleagues; the nurse may disagree with what the patient wishes and have to represent the patient to the team who do agree with the patient, and so on. Of course the answer to this exercise is to be found in the understanding that it is not what the nurse is advocating that is important – it is the fact that the nurse is acting as advocate which has moral relevance.

Activity 6.4 Reflection

Every day we consent to all manner of things without even noticing. We consent to allowing another person through a door ahead of us with a nod of the head; we consent to our car being serviced by the mechanic by taking it to the garage and we consent to the dentist undertaking a filling by opening our mouth! In the practice setting we witness consent in a variety of ways every day. This might range from a patient allowing us to use her first name to the patient holding out her arm so that we can take her blood pressure.

Activity 6.5 Critical thinking

The initial decision Frank made seemed to suit what he wanted and what he had come to terms with. The pressure from his family coerced him into changing his mind. This change of mind is probably not in Frank's best interests and is a direct response to the fact that the family do not understand what is going on and do not wish to lose their loved one. The response of the family is quite understandable. Here again the solution to the problem is to communicate with the family regarding the issues at stake, helping them understand the enormous burden of haemodialysis on Frank and how it may be in his best interests if he did not dialyse. Whatever the situation, it should be Frank's decision and he should be empowered to make a decision which he feels best fits what he wants to do. In reality it may be OK for Frank to be coerced by his family as he regards this as more important than standing by his original decision – of course, starting dialysis is not a one-way street and he may make the decision to withdraw at a later date once the family understand the negative impact of dialysis on his quality of life. If you meet similar situations in practice you will see they are very situational and you may wish to discuss the issues in each point of view with your tutor or mentor.

Activity 6.7 Communication

In this situation, the communication between Simon and Daniel is insufficient to allow Daniel to exercise free choice over what will happen to him. Simon has stifled any chance of Daniel making a free choice about what will happen to him since he has not provided him with any explanation of the alternatives. Ben should ask Simon to come back to the ward and ensure that Daniel has a full explanation regarding his options and their potential side effects before he is asked to make any choices. Should Ben not feel able to do this, he should raise the issue with his mentor, the ward sister or nurse-in-charge who, as trained nurses, would be accountable for acting on the information Ben had given them.

Further reading

Hansen, I (2004) An intercultural nursing perspective on autonomy. *Nursing Ethics*, 11(1): 28–41.
An interesting challenge to the usual thinking about autonomy in nursing.

Wertheimer, A and Miller, FG (2008) Payment for research participation: a coercive offer? *Journal of Medical Ethics*, 34: 389–392.
Quite a detailed, but fascinating, take on the question of paying research subjects.

Useful websites

www.bma.org.uk/advice/employment/ethics/medical-students-ethics-toolkit/6-consent-to-treatment-capacity
A guide to consent from the British Medical Association.

www.mind.org.uk/information-support/legal-rights/consent-to-treatment
A guide to consent from Mind, the mental health charity.

www.nhs.uk/Conditions/Consent-to-treatment/Pages/Introduction.aspx
A useful guide to consent from the NHS.

www.nmc-uk.org/Nurses-and-midwives/Regulation-in-practice/Regulation-in-Practice-Topics/consent/
A guide to consent from the Nursing and Midwifery Council.

www.rcn.org.uk/get-help/rcn-advice/consent
A guide to consent from the Royal College of Nursing.

Chapter 7
Dilemmas at the start and end of life

Peter Ellis and Hilary Engward

···
NMC Standards for Pre-registration Nursing Education

This chapter will address the following competencies:

Domain 1: Professional values

Generic standard for competence

1.   All nurses must practise with confidence according to *The Code: Professional Standards of Practice and Behaviour for Nurses and Midwives* (NMC, 2015), and within other recognised ethical and legal frameworks. They must be able to recognise and address ethical challenges relating to people's choices and decision making about their care, and act within the law to help them and their families and carers find acceptable solutions.

1.1. Adult nurses must understand and apply current legislation to all service users, paying special attention to the protection of vulnerable people, including those with complex needs arising from ageing, cognitive impairment, long-term conditions and those approaching the end of life.

3.   All nurses must support and promote the health, wellbeing, rights and dignity of people, groups, communities and populations. These include people whose lives are affected by ill health, disability, ageing, death and dying. Nurses must understand how these activities influence public health.

Domain 2: Communication and interpersonal skills

1.   All nurses must build partnerships and therapeutic relationships through safe, effective and non-discriminatory communication. They must take account of individual differences, capabilities and needs.

8.   All nurses must respect individual rights to confidentiality and keep information secure and confidential in accordance with the law and relevant ethical and regulatory frameworks, taking account of local protocols. They must also actively share personal information with others when the interests of safety and protection override the need for confidentiality.

Domain 4: Leadership, management and team working

6.   All nurses must work independently as well as in teams. They must be able to take the lead in coordinating, delegating and supervising care safely, managing risk and remaining accountable for the care given.
···

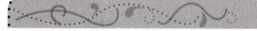

NMC Essential Skills Clusters

This chapter will address the following ESCs:

Care, compassion and communication
Patients/clients can trust a newly registered graduate nurse to:
2. Engage in person-centred care empowering people to make choices about how their needs are met when they are unable to meet them for themselves.
3. Respect them as individuals and strive to help them the preserve their dignity at all times.

Organisational aspects of care
Patients/clients can trust a newly registered graduate nurse to:
17. Work safely under pressure and maintain the safety of service users at all times.
19. Work to prevent and resolve conflict and maintain a safe environment.

Chapter aims

After reading this chapter you will be able to:

*   discuss the nature of dilemmas in healthcare;
*   identify strategies with which to address ethical dilemmas which arise in practice;
*   consider key ethical issues relating to abortion and euthanasia;
*   differentiate amongst various approaches to the moral status of the foetus and the dying adult.

Introduction

This chapter is unlike most of the other chapters in this book as, instead of looking at ethical concepts and how they might apply to a variety of clinical and practice issues, we will look at two ethical dilemmas and apply some ethical theories and concepts to them. We could have chosen any number of dilemmas with which to illustrate the process of decision making in dilemmatic situations but we have chosen to explore two of the most dramatic and contentious: abortion and euthanasia.

The reasons why we have chosen these topics is that they are serve to illustrate some of the principles, ideas and strategies we identify throughout the book. These issues are also timeless, in that they have tested ethical thought for centuries and are likely to continue to do so since both dilemmas are to some extent immediately impacted upon by changes in medical and nursing technology and research – that is to say, as knowledge changes so does the empirical evidence (see Chapter 8) underpinning the arguments around the beginning and end of life.

We have identified in this book that we ought to use ethical principles inductively to guide our thinking and decision making and we hope to be able to demonstrate this in action in this chapter. First of all we should start by considering what constitutes an ethical dilemma.

Ethical dilemmas

A dilemma arises in situations where the right course of action is not obvious. Dilemmas arise when we just do not know what to do for the best. Melia (2014) gives the example of not knowing who to save during a difficult birth, the mother or the baby. This is an example of a true moral dilemma since whichever way one acts there is a genuinely negative outcome for someone. One could spent a lot of time constructing ethical and moral arguments for one course of action or another and both would in all likelihood be right – and wrong.

Not all activity in life or nursing practice generates ethical dilemmas. This is perhaps best illustrated by thinking about the opposite scenario: where the ethical course of action is clear, when there are no ethically right alternative courses of action to choose from.

Scenario: doing the right thing

Nishie is a student nurse in her second year of training. While on placement on a medical ward Nishie is tasked with helping one of the care assistants with providing last offices to a recently dead patient in one of the side rooms. Nishie and the care assistant clear the dead patient's locker and account for all of her belongings, filling in the property book and placing the items in the ward safe. After returning to the patient and finishing providing last offices Nishie is alone for a moment with the patient. Nishie notices there is a £10 note in the top compartment of the locker. Nishie picks up the note and then goes to find the care assistant so that they can amend the property book and add the £10 to the property in the ward safe.

In this scenario, there is no dilemma since there is only one right thing to do: put the money with the rest of the deceased's possessions. All ethical schools of thought and principles would point in the direction of action which Nishie took. In reality for Nishie there were only two choices – do the right thing or steal.

Not all ethical issues are so clear-cut and as a result they require some considerable thought on our part as nurses. It is important for us to consider the various ethical and legal principles, social norms, facts and ideals which we can use to guide our decision making. These things, taken together with the idea of inductive thinking, guided by reflection on experience (as we discussed in Chapter 2), provide us with some powerful and useful tools with which to address ethical questions.

This chapter aims to analyse the important issues and arguments of both the abortion and euthanasia debates in such a way as to help us focus on the reasons underpinning the arguments as well as to determine the consistency of such arguments. The goal of this chapter is not to convince you to accept one position or the other, but to help you to understand some of the arguments which inform both sides as well as helping you to consider the manner in which reasonable debate might be formulated.

Abortion

Abortion has been legal in the UK since the Abortion Act 1967 (HM Government, 1967) as amended by the Human Fertilisation and Embryology Act 1990 (HM Government, 1990) which permits the termination of a pregnancy by a registered medical practitioner subject to certain conditions. In England, Scotland and Wales, abortion is provided free of charge if the woman is resident in the UK and entitled to NHS care.

Concept summary: UK law and abortion

The Abortion Act (HM Government, 1967) amended by the Human Fertilisation and Embryology Act (HM Government, 1990) applies to England, Scotland and Wales and indicates when an abortion may be legally carried out. The Act, as amended by section 37 of the Human Fertilisation and Embryology Act 1990, permits abortion when:

the pregnancy has not exceeded its twenty-fourth week and the continuance of the pregnancy would involve risk, greater than if the pregnancy were terminated, of injury of the physical or mental health of the woman or any existing children of her family.

This amendment introduced viability at the 24th week, reducing the limit from the prior 28 weeks in the Infant Life (Preservation) Act (HM Government, 1929). The reduction to 24 weeks reflected technological developments that enable survival outside the uterus at earlier stages of foetal development. Advances in medical science and technology will continue to push the boundaries of fetal viability and will require changes in legislation to reflect this in all likelihood.

Within the terms of the Abortion Act, only a registered practitioner can terminate a pregnancy and a legally induced abortion must be certified by two registered medical practitioners as justified under one or more of the following grounds:

A. *the continuance of the pregnancy would involve risk to the life of the pregnant woman greater than if the pregnancy were terminated (Abortion Act, 1967 as amended, section 1(1)(c))*
B. *the termination is necessary to prevent grave permanent injury to the physical or mental health of the pregnant woman (section 1(1)(b))*

(continued)

> *(continued)*
>
> C. the pregnancy has not exceeded its twenty-fourth week and that the continuance of the pregnancy would involve risk, greater than if the pregnancy were terminated, of injury to the physical or mental health of the pregnant woman (section 1(1)(a))
>
> D. the pregnancy has not exceeded its twenty-fourth week and that the continuance of the pregnancy would involve risk, greater than if the pregnancy were terminated, of injury to the physical or mental health of any existing children of the family of the pregnant woman (section 1(1)(a))
>
> E. there is a substantial risk that if the child were born it would suffer from such physical or mental abnormalities as to be seriously handicapped (section 1(1)(d)) or, in an emergency, certified by the operating practitioner as immediately necessary
>
> F. to save the life of the pregnant woman (section 1(4))
>
> G. to prevent grave permanent injury to the physical or mental health of the pregnant woman (section 1(4))
>
> **(www.gov.uk/government/uploads/system/uploads/attachment_data/ file/307650/Abortion_statistics__England_and_Wales.pdf)**

Framed as a medically sanctioned defence against a piece of criminal law passed in 1861, UK law could be viewed as out of step with contemporary society. Indeed, while women use abortion services in early pregnancy believing they have a right to make their own choice, British law still requires the identification of serious physical or mental health risk by two doctors not necessarily qualified in psychological disciplines, and there is broad consensus among practitioners that this is out of step with contemporary person centred health and medical practices. As such, UK abortion care providers appear to be seeking the liberalisation of Britain's abortion law that was passed 50 years ago, as reflected in the founding of a new support organisation for service providers, the British Society for Abortion Care Providers (BSACP) and a campaign for legal reform by the UK's largest service provider, the British Pregnancy Advisory Service (BPAS).

With the election of a pro-life president in the USA, and calls for the liberalisation of the Abortion Law in the UK, the abortion debate has never been more current. However, the central philosophical questions about abortion remain constant, those being tensions between women's right to self-determination about their bodies, and the ethical status and/or rights of the foetus. It also remains consistent for nurses to understand the basis of the abortion debate from the perspective of themselves as individual practitioners, from the perspective of the profession, and from the perspective of the individual woman.

Arguments about the ethical status of the foetus raise questions about issues such as 'can a foetus be considered to be a person?' and if it can, 'what moral status does it have'. Different perceptions within this debate are informed by cultural and religious ideologies about the status of the foetus and the position of women in society. The language used when discussing abortion can also be emotive or vague, for example, the terms **pro-life** and **pro-choice** are regularly used but do not tell us what counts as life and they tend not to consider the nuances of the individual's life when making a decision to terminate a pregnancy.

Framing the debate

How we think about the ethics of abortion depends on three main issues. First, there are *factual matters*, such as what happens at different stages of foetal development, and what the likely consequences are of certain actions given certain societal conditions. Second, there are the *ethical perspectives*, such as the nature and basis of moral rights. Third, there are conceptual matters, such as the meaning of terms such as abortion, personhood or human. Since these arguments interact and define the content of each other, they will be intertwined within the following discussion. Suffice to say, you should try to look out for each of the elements as we explore the ethical issues around abortion.

Factual, ethical and conceptual issues

Debate about abortion tends to focus on either the rights of women to **self-determination** over their bodies or the status accorded to the foetus. Generally there is a structure that underpins arguments for both cases.

The main arguments advanced against abortion:

- Premise A – the foetus is an innocent human being.
- Premise B – it is morally wrong to kill an innocent human being.
- Conclusion – it is morally wrong to kill a foetus.

This type of reasoning can also be used to support a pro-abortion point of view:

- Premise A – the foetus has no moral status.
- Premise B – it is not morally wrong to destroy something that has no moral status.
- Conclusion – it is not morally wrong to destroy a foetus.

Much of the debate in regard to abortion has centred around the first premise, whether or not the foetus is a person. If the foetus is a person, then does it have the same rights that belong to persons, including a right to life? So what we are really asking is what constitutes a person or personhood, and it is concepts of personhood that connect the foetus with a right to life.

Dealing with the conceptual matters present in an ethical argument is a bit like defining terms in an essay. For example if you were to write about the consequentialist view of abortion, you would have to define which consequences you were interested in (e.g. happiness, pain). You would also need to define what you mean by abortion, why and under what circumstances it was taking place. Unless other people involved in a debate understand what you mean by the terms you use then there is considerable room for misunderstanding.

Within the abortion debate there are considerable difficulties of definition and terminology, with proponents on both sides trying to grapple with some difficult ethical and philosophical concepts.

Concept summary: necessary/sufficient conditions

When thinking about what constitutes personhood, we think about what is needed, or necessary, and what is sufficient.

- A **necessary condition** is something which must be present for another thing to be possible, e.g. there must be air to support human life.
- A **sufficient condition** is something which, if present, provides sufficient grounds to believe something else is true, e.g. while air is certainly necessary for humans to live, it is not, by itself, sufficient.

Since the issue of whether or not a foetus is a person is so fundamental to debates on abortion, it is worth taking some time to explore what conditions are necessary, or sufficient, in order for something to be considered to be a person.

Activity 7.1 *Critical thinking*

Consider the following list. Which of these are *necessary* to constitute a person, and which are *sufficient*?

- conceived by humans;
- genetic structure;
- physical resemblance;
- presence of a soul;
- viability;
- having the potential to experience a future like ours.

There are some possible answers to all activities at the end of the chapter, unless otherwise indicated.

Arguments regarding abortion often hinge on the conceptual issue of what constitutes personhood. There are also debates that do not consider the moral status of the foetus. These arguments are typically based on utilitarian reasoning or on claims about the rights of persons. There are therefore two types of arguments for and against abortion:

1. arguments for which the moral status of the foetus is relevant;
2. arguments for which the moral status of the foetus is irrelevant.

To start with, we explore arguments which consider the moral status as relevant, followed by the second perspective, that the moral status is irrelevant.

Arguments that depend on the moral status of the foetus

Arguments that emphasise the moral status of the foetus ask a broad range of questions, such as:

- Is the foetus a person?
- Does a foetus have a moral value?
- If a foetus has a moral value, what type of value is this?
- Does the moral value of the foetus alter at differing stages of its development?
- If the moral value of a foetus changes over time, when do the key milestones happen?

These questions are **ontological** because they ask what sort of a being a foetus is, e.g. is it a being in its own right, or part of its mother? And, if the foetus is a being, what kind of moral worth might that confer upon it? They also pose a pivotal question about when the moral value of the foetus is such that it can be considered to be of the same, or at least very similar, worth to that of someone who has already been born.

There are two ways to try to answer this question. One way is to focus on the characteristics of the foetus and try to identify a point at which it has sufficient characteristics for it to be considered as a person worthy of moral concern. The other way is to ask what kind of beings, of any sort (human or non-human), have special moral status, such as the right to life.

The first way refers to foetal development and asks three questions about each developmental stage – these are both *factual* and *conceptual* questions. What characteristics are present in the developing foetus? When are these characteristics present? Why are these characteristics significant and why might they confer special moral status?

The first two of these points can be considered by looking at the stages of foetal development. At approximately week 2 post-conception, the embryo embeds in the uterus wall; during weeks 2–8 organ systems such as the brain and the heart develop; at weeks 20–26 the ability to sense pain develops and at week 40 the baby is born. Changes in foetal development are gradual and bring with them different understandings about the status of the foetus. Whilst these changes do not in themselves lead to ethical conclusions, they do provide a standard framework for any discussion about foetal development.

The third point considers what is significant at any point in foetal development, and how this confers some kind of moral status. To explore this, we need to consider what it means to be human.

Activity 7.2 — *Critical thinking*

Mary is 20-weeks' pregnant and is requesting a termination of pregnancy. There are no known abnormalities of the foetus; however, Mary is concerned she cannot cope with the baby. What moral and ethical arguments might be pertinent to this request? Do you think a termination of a 20-week foetus is permissible?

Being human

The argument here is that human foetuses are members of the human race and therefore have equal moral value with all other human beings. The argument is: 'all human beings have moral worth' – it is the biological determination of *being human* that is important.

Concept summary: the argument about human worth

- All humans have worth.
- The foetus is a human at some stage in its development.
- The foetus has **human worth** at some defined point.

If the argument about abortion hinges on the notion of when a foetus becomes a human, or that there is something important about human biology, then we can start to see the difficulties which the abortion debate suffers from. For example, it could be argued that unfertilised eggs/sperm are biologically human; however, most people do not consider them to have specific moral worth as human beings.

Questions can also be asked about why only humans are included here. If other species are sufficiently like us in relevant aspects, then should they be considered as having the same moral worth as humans? In considering this, we are questioning whether it is membership of a species which determines moral worth. It may therefore be that we are asking what it is to be human, or *being like human.*

If what is ethically relevant is *being like human* then questions about what characteristics of *being like human* are significant enough to confer moral status need to be asked. Arguments about the ability to communicate and reason are often cited but, for these to work, we need to answer questions about how we differentiate these characteristics in humans from those in other animal species such as the great apes. Also what does this argument mean for humans who lack the capacity to communicate or reason? Do they have no, or lower, moral value? Is someone's moral worth then directly proportional to his or her ability to communicate and to reason?

This line of thought leads us to the notion that it is merely membership of the species which might prove the determinant of moral worth. If any human has the requisite status, then we all do, regardless of what we are like or what capacities we possess.

Other activists in the abortion debate regard this ideology as being too simplistic and suggest that it cannot be just the species we belong to but the individual capacities we have, as a species, which are important. The question is then: when do these characteristics start to have value?

- When there is a possibility of developing the characteristic (**potentiality**)?
- When the characteristic is evolving?
- When the characteristic has fully developed (**actuality**)?

Potentiality

This position considers that all beings that have power to develop certain key characteristics have moral worth. Therefore, if a foetus has the potential to develop the requisite moral capacities, the foetus has moral worth. Following this argument, abortion is wrong because it prevents a being from *actualising* (that is, actually achieving its potential). However, a foetus that does not possess this potential, e.g. an **anencephalic** foetus, does not have the same status.

Potentiality is a powerful argument. However, it does not answer the question as to whether it is being aware of potentiality or simply having potentiality which is important. For example, is it possible to deprive someone of something that person is not conscious of having? If a foetus is unaware of its potentiality to develop into a future person and is aborted, has it been deprived of anything?

Tooley (1972) forwards the following analogy to help us think this through. Suppose we have a kitten that will mature into a cat if left alone. We also have a serum that if injected into the kitten will make it grow into a human being. Tooley suggests that there is little reason to allow the kitten to develop into a human, since although it has potential to develop into one post-injection, it is not yet actually a human. Tooley (1972) concludes:

> *if it is seriously wrong to kill something, the reason cannot be that it will later acquire properties that in themselves provide something with a right to life … if it is wrong to kill a human foetus, it cannot be because of potentialities.*

Tooley's point is that those *potentialities* are merely *potentialities*, and are as yet not *actual* and therefore cannot be afforded significance.

Actuality

If we cannot rely on potentiality to develop certain characteristics, then maybe we should consider what is actually present. The argument of actuality considers the presence of certain characteristics as sufficient to gain moral worth. This refers us back to the consideration of which characteristics carry moral weight. For example, if high-level characteristics, say reasoning and communication, are valued, then a newborn would not necessarily be included.

The philosopher Mary Anne Warren (1973) writes that, although the foetus, newborn and young child are humans biologically, they are not yet persons or beings with requisite moral status. There may be good reasons to treat them well, but it is not necessarily because they are *persons* with rights.

Evolving value

The intermediate position between potentiality and actuality is that of evolving value. This position contends that *potential* counts but not as much as *actual* possession of certain characteristics. As the potential is realised, moral status is also given. Applying the criterion to foetal development, the early-term foetus has less moral worth than the late-term foetus. This approach parallels the legal approach in that termination of pregnancy can legally occur up to 24 weeks' gestation.

Arguments for which the moral status of the foetus is irrelevant

Utilitarian reasoning

Utilitarian arguments about abortion tend to refer to the potential consequences of a continued pregnancy, e.g. loss of job/opportunities for the woman or suffering of the future person.

Using act utilitarian reasoning (see Chapter 4), each instance of abortion stands on its own with regard to determining whether the abortion is a good or bad thing. Consequences to consider include: physical health risks and benefits; positive or negative mental consequences; and financial and social outcomes. Note that whether the foetus is a person is not among the issues being considered when arguing from this perspective.

From a utilitarian or consequentialist perspective, abortion is sometimes morally permissible and sometimes not: it would depend on the consequences. Good moral judgements about abortion will depend on the adequacy of the prediction of consequences. Critics of the act utilitarian argument object to its disregard of rights and point out that this may condone the taking of any life if the overall consequences of doing so are favourable.

A rule utilitarian (see Chapter 4) would consider which practice regarding abortion would be best for society as a whole, e.g. would the rule 'no one should have an abortion' be likely to maximise happiness? Or perhaps the rule 'no one should have an abortion unless the pregnancy threatens the mother's health or wellbeing' is more likely to have better overall consequences? The important thing here is: what action would as a rule produce the best outcomes for society on the whole?

Rights arguments

An influential argument about the rights of persons that does not consider the moral status of the foetus as relevant is that forwarded by Judith Jarvis Thomson (1971) and later added to by Jane English (1984). Thomson argues that, even if the foetus could be considered a person, abortion may be morally justified. In other words, she challenges the premise that it is always wrong to end the life of another. To make her case, Thomson, for the sake of argument, assumes the foetus does have moral status from early in pregnancy, but poses the question as to whether the pregnant woman has an obligation to sustain the life of the foetus by providing it with the use of her body.

To explore this, Thomson puts forward an analogy where you imagine yourself waking up to find yourself attached to a famous violinist through various medical devices and tubes. You are told that you have been kidnapped and hooked up to the violinist to keep him alive. The question Thomson poses is: would you be morally justified in unplugging yourself from the violinist, even though doing so would result in the death of the violinist? Thomson argues that you would be justified in doing so because you have not consented to using your body to save the violinist's life.

The concept of consent here is used to refer to a deliberate or planned choice (see Chapter 6), where although it may be generous for you to save the life of the violinist (or the foetus), you are not obligated to do so. The point here is that no one has the right to use someone's body for any purpose, unless given permission to do so.

Thomson's analogy has several limitations in that it mainly refers to cases of pregnancy following rape, and the violinist has no potential relationship to you. Thomson's analogy remains useful because it does provide a good argument to justify abortion for pregnancy following rape. The main point, Thomson argues, is that it is the woman's right to choose whether to allow her body to be used or not, whether in the case of rape or accidental/unwanted pregnancy. The argument does not apply if sex has been consented in full knowledge of the potential consequences.

The philosopher Jane English (1984) amended Thomson's example to bring it more in line with conventional cases of unwanted pregnancy, using the following analogy. Imagine that you go out knowing that you might be rendered unconscious and hooked up to the violinist. You would still, according to English, be entitled to unhook yourself. This case is more closely analogous to conventional cases of unwanted pregnancies.

These utilitarian and rights-based arguments are examples of positions about abortion that do not depend on understandings of the moral status of the foetus.

Abortion conclusions

The arguments considered in this section of the chapter have questioned if and how moral status can be inferred to the foetus. If the foetus is considered as not having moral status, then abortion is possibly morally permissible. If it is considered to be a person, then abortion is morally problematic. If the foetus is said to have an in-between status, then conclusions may be dependent on the stage of development of the foetus. These arguments therefore stem from ideas about what moral status the foetus is said to have. However, as the utilitarian and rights-based arguments exemplify, there are other considerations, such as potential consequences for the woman and society, to be considered.

Finally, it is worth noting that something considered 'immoral' is not necessarily illegal. For example, if abortion were thought, for whatever reason, to be immoral, further reasons would need to be given to make it illegal. At the same time, we have to ask whether the only reason to make something illegal is if it is immoral. We may wish to permit people to make choices about morally problematic concerns and not interfere with this by imposing laws. This tends to be reflected when those who think abortion is morally wrong also believe that women ought to be permitted to make decisions about abortion based on their own conception of morality.

Considerations of abortion therefore may create any number of dilemmas for the nurse who knows that abortion is legal but may, or may not, believe abortion to be agreeable. Nurses and midwives do not have the right to refuse to take part in any emergency treatment in any circumstances; however, there may be occasions when nurses and midwives have a conscientious objection to a particular aspect of patient care. Whilst the Nursing and Midwifery Council (NMC) expects nurses and midwives at all times to adhere to the principles contained within *The Code: Professional Standards of Practice and Behaviour for Nurses and Midwives* (NMC, 2015), in law they do have the right to object conscientiously in two areas only.

Article 4(1) of the Abortion Act 1967 (Scotland, England and Wales)

This provision gives nurses and midwives with a conscientious objection a qualified right to refuse to participate in the process of treatment where termination of pregnancy is the object.

Under section 4(1) no person who has a conscientious objection to participating in any activity governed by this Act shall be under any duty, however arising, to do so.

This right to conscientious objection is qualified by section 4(2) of the Act where it is made clear that nothing in subsection (1) shall affect any duty to participate in treatment which is necessary to save the life or prevent grave permanent injury to the physical or mental health of a pregnant woman.

In any legal proceedings the burden of proof of conscientious objection shall rest on the person claiming to rely on it.

Article 38(2) of the Human Fertilisation and Embryology Act 2008

This Act gives nurses and midwives the right to refuse to participate in technological procedures to achieve conception and pregnancy.

(www.nmc-uk.org/Nurses-and-midwives/Regulation-in-practice/Regulation-in-Practice-Topics/Conscientious-objection-by-nurses-and-midwives-/)

The NMC expects all nurses and midwives to be non-judgemental when providing care and to continue to provide service users with full, unbiased information related to their care. Nurses and midwives are expected to facilitate patient access to relevant healthcare services, including where termination of pregnancy may result, regardless of whether they have a conscientious objection.

Euthanasia

The makings of a dilemma

From a purely legal point of view there is nothing dilemmatic about euthanasia; it is illegal to aid a suicide in the UK and therefore euthanasia is something nurses should not engage in. The word euthanasia is derived from the Greek *eu* (good) and *thanatos* (death) and therefore literally means 'good death'. Euthanasia is a contentious topic in the UK, with various individuals and organisations taking a stance about it depending on their theological, philosophical or experiential position.

Before continuing to explore what euthanasia is and the arguments around it, in its various forms, it is worth considering why it might be considered to constitute an ethical dilemma. Remember, an ethical dilemma is a situation in which there are two or more options for action, each of which appears to be equally ethically right. At its simplest, arguments about euthanasia are between individuals who say it is always wrong to take a human life and those who claim that it is cruel to prolong life when an individual is in pain or suffering indignity – the dilemma being to continue to allow suffering or not by means of being involved in the taking of the life of another human being.

On immediate face value, there is nothing wrong with either argument. Taking a life is usually wrong; it violates most of the ethical principles contained within any ethical school of thought. For the consequentialist allowing the taking of lives causes a state of fear and therefore reduces overall happiness; the deontologist would normally follow the rule 'thou shall not kill' while for virtuous people the taking of another's life would not even feature in their thinking.

Conversely, the consequentialist would not support continued suffering as this reduces overall happiness (both for the individual and others who think that they may also be allowed to suffer at a later date); the deontologist might consider allowing suffering to violate the principles of 'doing good' and 'avoiding harm' while for the virtuous person allowing someone to suffer is anathema.

So here we are left with a confusing picture of what is ethical and what is not: this is a true ethical dilemma. The rest of this section will define and explore the issues arising from the various forms euthanasia might take and, in doing so, as with the earlier section on abortion, will perhaps provide you with ideas about how to think through different ethical dilemmas you might come across in practice.

Definitions of euthanasia

In this chapter we will define six classifications of euthanasia and discuss the details of each type. Understanding what we mean by euthanasia both from the point of view of what actions it entails and the participation in decision making of the individual to whom the euthanasia applies is important in trying to establish its ethicality, or not.

Classically euthanasia occurs in one of two ways. The first approach to euthanasia is what is termed passive. In **passive euthanasia** no one does anything directly to bring about the death of

119

the individual. Passive euthanasia implies that an individual is allowed to die even though that person's life might have been prolonged.

Case study: passive euthanasia: Tony Bland

*Tony Bland suffered severe brain damage when he was caught in serious overcrowding at the Hillsborough football stadium in 1989. Tony was left in what was termed a **persistent vegetative state** – a coma-like condition from which it was believed no one ever recovers.*

His doctors and parents were of the opinion that to all intents and purposes he was dead and applied to the courts to be allowed to:

- *discontinue all life-sustaining treatments, including ventilation, nutrition and hydration by artificial means;*
- *provide only treatment for the sole purpose of enabling him to end his life in dignity and free from pain and suffering;*
- *consider his death, as a result of the withdrawal/withholding of treatment, to be natural;*
- *protect the staff from any criminal or civil liability.*

Since Tony was not actively ventilated it was the withdrawal of medically supported feeding and hydration that led to his death from kidney failure. As nothing active had been done to bring about Tony's death this might be considered by some to be an example of passive euthanasia (Ellis, 1992).

The second form of euthanasia is termed active. In **active euthanasia** something is actively done to bring about the death of the individual. Active euthanasia implies that an individual's death is brought about earlier than it might have naturally occurred.

As we saw in Chapter 4 (see Concept Summary: Omission, commission and intent), there is often no ethical difference between an act of commission (e.g. active euthanasia) and an act of omission (e.g. passive euthanasia): what is important is the intention with which the act is pursued. When we follow this line of argument later in the chapter we will see that sometimes there appears to be a practical, normative, difference between the two.

Activity 7.3   *Reflection*

Think back to a time when you were involved in the care of a dying patient. What care was provided to the person and what care was stopped? Why was this?

As well as being either active or passive, euthanasia is defined in relation to the voluntariness of participation of the person to whom the euthanasia applies. There are three levels of voluntariness: voluntary, involuntary and non-voluntary. **Voluntary euthanasia** is said to occur when the individual requests to be euthanised; **involuntary euthanasia** occurs when the individual cannot participate in the decision (for example, because of dementia or because s/he is in a coma) and **non-voluntary euthanasia** is against the person's will.

Because of the nature of non-voluntary euthanasia, which is essentially murder, we will discount it from our further discussions. There is little which might be positively said about non-voluntary euthanasia since examples of it are exclusively associated with some of the most heinous of crimes. The unethical nature of non-voluntary euthanasia applies whether the death is achieved by active or passive means; an act of commission or omission.

Case study: non-voluntary euthanasia

During the Second World War in Nazi Germany, many people with learning difficulties and mental illness were killed in a programme called Action T4. The purpose of this state-sponsored euthanasia was to provide 'mercy deaths' to persons considered as 'incurables'.

Involuntary euthanasia refers to euthanasia applied to people who are not able to express, and have not previously expressed, a wish to die. The case of Tony Bland (see the earlier case study) is an example of this. There are, therefore, parallel ethical issues to consider when debating euthanasia: its voluntariness and the nature of the action required to achieve it. In the case of Tony Bland, the euthanasia in question was **involuntary passive euthanasia** – that is, he was unable to be involved in the decision making and his death was achieved by an act of omission.

Concept summary: definitions of types of euthanasia

	Voluntary	Involuntary
Passive	Voluntary passive	Involuntary passive
Active	Voluntary active	Involuntary active

Now we have identified the forms which euthanasia might take, we should explore some of the arguments for and against it, taking into account that euthanasia is seen by many people to constitute an ethical dilemma.

The argument about suffering

Of the arguments about euthanasia, the most frequently heard is that which touches on the emotive issues of human suffering. Suffering is hard to define and therefore the arguments which rely on it are both ill defined and contentious.

Consideration of the arguments about euthanasia from the point of view of suffering often divides people down one of two lines: those who say suffering can be managed and those who say it cannot. What probably divides the camps is agreeing on a definition of what constitutes suffering.

Physical pain is a frequent issue in terminal illness and therefore the management of pain is a priority. Those in favour of euthanasia often claim we are unable to manage all physical pain, especially in the terminally ill, while those against euthanasia cite the incredible work undertaken within the hospice movement as pointing to the fact that pain can be managed.

In a similar manner to the debate about abortion, which is impacted as technology changes the factual elements of the debate by reducing the age of viability, arguments about the management of pain will doubtless ebb and flow in response to the progress of pain management technologies. Arguments about suffering which rely on discussions of pain may miss the point: not all suffering is about pain. Many proponents of euthanasia, including those who seek it for themselves, identify issues around the inability to self-care, reduced quality of life, reliance on others and impacts of illness on personal dignity as important forms of suffering (Rietjens et al., 2009). In this way the argument reflects the issues discussed in relation to experiential and critical interests discussed in Chapter 5 and, as in that chapter, where people stand in relation to the argument about suffering depends to some extent on what they believe about the importance of different forms of interests.

Right to die/pro-choice

If we accept, at least in part, some of the arguments made in Chapter 5 about protection from suffering providing one good reason for the existence of rights, then there does appear to be a **prima facie** (initially plausible) justification for what might be called a **right to die**.

Again, thinking back to Chapter 5, we saw some rights operate as liberties; that is, they require other people to leave us alone. If the right to die is a liberty, then it requires that other people, often doctors and nurses, do not intervene to save (or perhaps prolong) our lives against our will. This simple interpretation of the operation of the *right to die* reflects what happens day in and day out in various care settings where life-sustaining care is either not started or is withdrawn.

Activity 7.4   *Research and critical thinking*

Go online and find the Assisted Dying Bill which went before the UK Parliament in 2015. Read the content and identify the strategies within the bill (which was rejected) which attempted to make sure the euthanasia would be what the person wanted and that they were of sound mind.

Where the right-to-die argument becomes more contentious is where the arguments suggest that it is a positive claim right; that is, a right which requires someone else actively to do something

discussion still holds it to be of value to him or her and where this is not the case, whether that person has capacity (see Chapter 6) and whether there is something we can do by way of an intervention to change this view.

Double effect

One of the challenges of caring for the dying is the fact that often the care we provide as nurses plays a role in foreshortening life. For instance, the management of terminal pain using opiates can, and does, further suppress the respiratory centres in the brain of the terminal patient, thus hastening death. This can both feel right, in managing the pain, but wrong in that it shortens life.

Activity 7.6   *Decision making*

You are in placement on an oncology ward providing care for a group of adults with varying severity of disease. One of the patients, Adebayo, is terminally ill and in the last days of her life. Adebayo has end-stage lung cancer and is struggling to breathe. Adebayo is very tired from making prolonged respiratory effort and is also in pain as a result of the spread of cancer to her bones. You enter the side room where Adebayo is being nursed and notice that she is quite agitated but that she is making little respiratory effort. Her family are clearly upset by what is happening. Your mentor suggests that the right thing to do is to give her another dose of the morphine she has been prescribed. Taking you aside, your mentor explains that the morphine will settle Adebayo, but that it may also stop her breathing; how do you feel about this?

In this scenario you are being asked to do something which may hasten death, but which also treats the symptoms of disease – in this case agitation probably associated with pain. The doctrine of double effect, from Roman Catholic teachings, is used in helping to explain and justify the negative side effects of some actions which people undertake in the care of others. It helps to explain why we feel that managing pain at the end of life which simultaneously speeds up death is not a bad thing.

Concept summary: conditions on the doctrine of double effect

- The act must be at least morally indifferent or good.
- The act is undertaken only willing the positive outcome.
- The good effect must not be a result of the bad effect.
- The act is undertaken for an important reason.

(Sulmasy and Pellegrino, 1999)

Thinking about double effect helps us as nurses come to terms with some of the negative impacts of what we provide in the way of care, especially in relation to the end of life, regardless of our position on the rightness or wrongness of euthanasia. The argument is simple: if we administer pain relief to a terminal patient with a view to managing the pain and death ensues as a result, then what we intended to do was right. This may help us live with scenarios such as that which applied to Adebayo.

Unlike the previous arguments about euthanasia, this is purely a practical response to the realities of terminal care.

Euthanasia conclusions

The arguments presented in this brief overview of some of the issues contained within the euthanasia debate demonstrate that the ethical dilemma surrounding the rightness or wrongness of euthanasia is quite complex. This complexity is manifested in some of the definitions of euthanasia, which in themselves change the manner in which the arguments can be pursued, as well as in recognising the very personal nature of some of the interpretations of reasons for euthanasia.

As an ethical subject matter, euthanasia is likely to remain contentious, with arguments on both sides having considerable ethical, legal and logical weight. Like abortion, however, the ethicality of euthanasia, or not, has to play second fiddle to its legality. In terms of action then there is no real dilemma for the nurse; in terms of whether the inability to provide active euthanasia is ethically correct, that is a matter for considerable debate.

Chapter summary

The main purpose of this chapter has been to allow you to see how some of the arguments about different ethical issues and dilemmas are constructed. It has illustrated that ethical thinking and principles can be used to construct arguments which can be used to inform ethical thought and decision making. A further message you might take from this chapter is that ethical thought might not always provide an answer to a situation and therefore there is a need for nurses to become comfortable with some aspects of greyness in their practice. This is not to say we abandon our values and principles, rather that they flex and change as a result of experience, reflection (see Chapter 2) and in the face of difficult clinical scenarios.

Abortion and euthanasia are stark examples of ethical issues which face healthcare providers. There are many other issues which face nurses and other healthcare professionals on a day-to-day basis in the care setting and any one of these might equally have been explored usefully in this chapter. We hope that by considering the arguments and counter-arguments that you can see how the debates about ethical issues of interest are constructed.

Activities: brief outline answers

Activity 7.1 Critical thinking

This activity asked to consider what is essential to constitute a person. Here there is likely to be only one necessary condition to constitute being a person, that being genetic structure. The others may be sufficient, but not absolutely necessary. For example, being conceived by humans could refer to human genetic material being used to aid in vitro conception; however becoming human will only occur with human genetic material. Viability may be a necessary condition; however, it could be argued that those that lack viability to survive independently have less personhood (e.g. an anencephalic baby). Other considerations, such as physical resemblance, presence of a soul, having potential to have a future like ours, may be considered as sufficient and important, but not absolutely necessary.

Activity 7.2 Critical thinking

This case requires us to think about the concepts of sentience and viability. These two issues are not the same but will be considered together because they occur approximately at the same time, around 20–24 weeks of gestation. Sentience refers to the foetus's ability to feel and experience pain. Viability is the foetus's ability to survive outside the uterus.

Sentience is a morally significant criterion as it denotes a being's ability to have meaningful experiences, and to have developed an interest for its own wellbeing. In addition to establishing the moral limits of aborting human foetuses, the argument from sentience is also deployed to defend animal rights.

Viability is considered a morally important point because it signifies the time where the human foetus can survive as an independent human being, without the assistance of its mother's body.

The UK law recognises the moral importance of viability, and stipulates the 24th week as the limit of elective abortion under section 1(1)(a) of the Abortion Act. The implications of this are that abortion prior to the point at which a foetus becomes sentient or viable is morally unproblematic. Abortion after this point is not permissible. It is therefore permissible for Mary to have a termination of pregnancy.

Activity 7.3 Reflection

This is quite a challenging issue to think about, but it is important that nurses learn to talk about and understand issues at the end of life. Just because someone is at the end of life does not mean we usually withdraw all care. For example, we provide pain relief, sedation and hydration and try to maintain the person's comfort and personal hygiene. We might stop medication for other things such as blood pressure or cholesterol management; this is just good sense.

For student nurses trying to make sense of this process it is worth discussing the feelings you have with your mentor and lecturers. What you should identify is that *not for cure* does not mean *not for care* and that since dying is a natural part of the cycle of life, care of the dying should feel *right* and part of what we do as nursing professionals. Allowing someone to die and maintaining that person's comfort at the end of life can, and should, be a positive experience.

Activity 7.4 Research and critical thinking

The Bill recognises some of the pitfalls of introducing euthanasia: it includes the need for the disease to be terminal and the person in the last six months of life; the need for a second doctor; the need for the person to have capacity; the provision for the person to withdraw from the arrangement at any time.

Activity 7.5 Critical thinking

The appeal of the concept of pro-life, especially to nurses, lies, at least in part, within the notion that we enter the profession to make people's lives better. Without life there are no lives to make better. We value life also because we spend much of our training and working lives trying to save lives and therefore death and dying are anathema to us.

Activity 7.6 Decision making

This is a fairly common scenario and is in some senses a pragmatic response to an issue which the UK has not legislated for. Clearly there are two key emotions at play here: the first says we need to deal with the pain and distress and the other that we should not take a life. It is very right to experience a mix of emotional responses to this scenario as this represents a proper human response as well as ethical and moral awareness. If you felt nothing it would be a cause for concern! It is right and proper in such scenarios that you should discuss what has happened and what you feel about it with your mentor, peers and university tutor. Rationalising such scenarios feels almost wrong, but is a right and proper way of us protecting ourselves emotionally as well as engaging with our humane nursing nature.

Further reading

Allmark, P, Cobb, M, Liddle, BJ and Tod, A (no date) *Is the Doctrine of Double Effect Irrelevant in End-of-Life Decision Making?* Available online at: http://shura.shu.ac.uk/2341/2/NP_Resubmission_DDE_%232.pdf (accessed 30/12/16).

A very interesting discussion about the doctrine of double effect.

Hurst, L (2005) The legal landscape at the threshold of viability for extremely premature infants: a nursing perspective, part 1. *Journal of Prenatal and Neonatal Nursing*, 19(2): 155–166.

Hursthouse, R (1987) *Beginning Lives.* Oxford: Basil Blackwell.

The classic text about the ethics of abortion.

Quaghebeur, T, Dierckx de Casterlé, B and Gastmans, C (2009) Nursing and euthanasia: a review of argument-based ethics literature. *Nursing Ethics*, 16(4): 466–486.

A good review of the existing literature in this area.

Regan, T (ed.) (1992) *Matters of Life and Death: New Introductory Essays in Moral Philosophy*, 3rd edn. London: McGraw-Hill.

A really good read with some of the world's best thinkers on this subject matter.

Shaw, AB (2002) Two challenges to the double effect doctrine: euthanasia and abortion. *Journal of Medical Ethics*, 28: 102–104.

A useful look into this subject from both the abortion and euthanasia viewpoint.

Steinbock, B (1996) *Life before Birth.* New York: Oxford University Press.

One of the best-known philosophical texts on abortion.

Useful websites

bma.org.uk/practical-support-at-work/ethics/ethics-a-to-z
Index for British Medical Association guidance on ethical issues.

www.wetrustwomen.org.uk/
The British Pregnancy Advisory Service (BPAS) 'We Trust Women' campaign website.

https://bsacp.org.uk/
The British Society for Abortion Care Providers (BSACP) website.

www.carenotkilling.org.uk

The website of Care Not Killing, a campaigning society which is anti-euthanasia.

www.dignityindying.org.uk

The website of Dignity in Dying, a campaigning society which is pro-euthanasia.

www.mariestopes.org.uk

The website of Marie Stopes, sexual healthcare and abortion provider.

www.nhs.uk/conditions/Abortion/Pages/Introduction.aspx

The NHS Choices website about abortion.

www.rcn.org.uk/__data/assets/pdf_file/0004/529654/Termination_of_pregnancy_WEB.pdf

The Royal College of Nursing's framework on abortion provision.

www.spuc.org.uk

The Society for Protection of Unborn Children (SPUC) affirms, defends and promotes the existence and value of human life from the moment of conception.

Chapter 8
Your ethical future

Hilary Engward

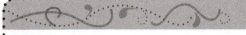

NMC Standards for Pre-registration Nursing Education

This chapter will address the following competencies:

Domain 1: Professional values

1. All nurses must practise with confidence according to *The Code: Professional Standards of Practice and Behaviour for Nurses and Midwives* (NMC, 2015). They must be able to recognise and address ethical challenges relating to people's choices and decision making about their care, and act within the law to help them and their families and carers find acceptable solutions.

7. All nurses must be responsible and accountable for keeping their knowledge and skills up to date through continuing professional development. They must aim to improve their performance and enhance the safety and quality of care through evaluation, supervision and appraisal.

Domain 2: Communication and interpersonal skills

1. All nurses must build partnerships and therapeutic relationships through safe, effective and non-discriminatory communication. They must take account of individual differences, capabilities and needs.

Domain 4: Leadership, management and team working

2. All nurses must be self-aware and recognise how their own values, principles and assumptions may affect their practice. They must maintain their own personal and professional development, learning from experience, through supervision, feedback, reflection and evaluation.

NMC Essential Skills Clusters

This chapter will address the following ESCs:

Care, compassion and communication

2. People can trust the newly qualified graduate nurse to engage in person-centred care, empowering people to make choices about how their needs are met when they are unable to meet them themselves.

3. People can trust the newly qualified graduate nurse to respect them as individuals and strive to help them preserve their dignity at all times.

> ## Chapter aims
>
> After reading this chapter, you will be able to:
>
> * explain what ethical practice is;
> * understand why ethical practice might not always occur;
> * know what is meant by the duty of candour;
> * explore how you might inquire into aspects of ethical practice at the local level;
> * identify the challenges that lie ahead for you as an ethically active nurse.

Introduction

The purpose of this chapter is to explore how ethics is useful to nurses and nursing students in the everyday practice of healthcare work, and to consider how we can contribute to the develop of organisations which are inherently ethical. The second important aim of this chapter is to help you consider how you might take what you have learnt in this book forward with you into your nursing career. To do this, the concepts of ethical leadership, and the duty of **candour** and **empirical ethics**, will be explored.

The Francis Report (2013), an independent public inquiry into poor standards of care at the Mid Staffordshire NHS Foundation Trust, detailed failings in the central aspects of nursing care: for example, failure to hydrate and feed patients, failure to respect privacy and dignity and a lack of compassion. This was compounded by a management culture that valued financially driven care targets over patient care, a lack of a 'caring and compassionate' culture and also a discouragement of staff expressing concerns about poor standards of care. The likelihood is that no one health professional at Mid Staffs intended this to occur, but it did. The important question to ask therefore is: how did health professionals allow this to happen? How did the healthcare professionals not act in accordance with their duty to care for and protect their patients from harm? If staff knew what was happening was wrong, why did they not do something about it?

Of course, we can't assume that all healthcare professionals in Mid Staffs were unaware of the differences between what was occurring and what ought to occur, nor that all professionals lacked the intrinsic characteristics to be an ethical practitioner; however, neglect did occur. Central to considering these issues and what they mean for caring professionals in general, and nurses in particular, are the wider structures within which individual practitioners work: the culture of the healthcare organisation and the type and style of leadership within that organisation.

The ethicality of organisations may seem to lie outside the remit of the student nurse. However, as an individual working within organisations with the duty to promote good and prevent intentional harms towards others, it is an essential area of understanding all nurses need to develop. Leadership is an important feature of the Nursing and Midwifery Council (NMC) *Standards for Pre-registration Nursing Education* (NMC, 2010), as can be seen at the start of the chapter.

Leadership responsibility for nurses, and nursing students, starts immediately when they start working in any care environment and the duties which attend this responsibility – including that of protection of the public at large – are clearly laid out in the NMC *Code* for nurses and midwives (2015). In particular:

16 Act without delay if you believe that there is a risk to patient safety or public protection

To achieve this, you must:

16.1 raise and, if necessary, escalate any concerns you may have about patient or public safety, or the level of care people are receiving in your workplace or any other healthcare setting and use the channels available to you in line with our guidance and your local working practices

16.2 raise your concerns immediately if you are being asked to practise beyond your role, experience and training

16.3 tell someone in authority at the first reasonable opportunity if you experience problems that may prevent you working within the Code or other national standards, taking prompt action to tackle the causes of concern if you can.

What is clear, therefore, is that developing awareness of our wider duties as ethical practitioners, leaders and contributors to organisations is not confined to the period following qualification, but that it is something we need to prepare for from the moment we enter the nursing profession as students.

Duty of candour

Activity 8.1   *Decision making*

Ruth is on a clinical placement on a unit for people with dementia in a care home. Ruth witnesses two care assistants 'manhandling' a patient into bed. Later she becomes aware that the patient has some bruising on her arm as a result of their treatment. Ruth is concerned about both the manual handling and the bruising and has to make a decision about what she will do about both: should she keep quiet or should she say something?

There are some possible answers to all activities at the end of the chapter, unless otherwise indicated.

Activity 8.1 is a common scenario: here the harm is not deliberate but nevertheless there is harm done and this needs to be addressed. One of the key issues raised here is about the need for Ruth to consider the ethicality of not acting on what she has seen.

Here the duty of candour is important, but is not always clearly understood by nurses. For example, when applying for registration or seeking renewal of registration with the NMC, nurses and midwives are required to sign a self-declaration. The self-declaration covers an intention to comply with the entirety of *The Code* and to be open and honest and act with integrity. *The Code* also places a clear obligation on nurses and midwives to act without delay if they believe that they, a colleague or anyone else may be putting someone at risk. They are also under a duty to raise concerns if they experience problems that prevent them from working within *The Code* or if problems in the care environment are putting patients at risk – all issues we see reflected in the student guidance.

The statutory duty of candour arose directly from the Francis Report (2013) which called for openness and transparency in the NHS to prevent a repeat of the deliberate concealment of poor care and negligence. This led to Regulation 20: duty of candour which defines what constitutes a notifiable safety incident for health and social care providers, specifically paragraph 8 which defines harm thresholds that trigger the duty of candour. Although Regulation 20 applies to organisations, rather than individual members of staff, it does require all health and social care organisations to ensure that all staff, regardless of level or permanency, understand the organisation's responsibility to be honest and transparent. In short, regulation 20 stipulates that organisations need to have policies and procedures that support a culture of openness and transparency, and that staff understand and follow these policies and procedures. This also includes action against bullying, harassment and undermining of staff who exercise their duty of candour.

In addition, all registered nurses are subject to the professional duty of candour, as overseen by the NMC. The professional duty of candour is explicit in *The Code*, section 14: be open and candid with all service users about all aspects of care and treatment, including when any mistakes or harm have taken place:

14.1 act immediately to put right the situation if someone has suffered actual harm for any reason or an incident has happened which had the potential for harm

14.2 explain fully and promptly what has happened, including the likely effects, and apologise to the person affected and, where appropriate, their advocate, family or carers, and

14.3 document all these events formally and take further action (escalate) if appropriate so they can be dealt with quickly.

The NMC have created guidance collaboratively with the GMC because healthcare is often provided by teams of doctors, nurses and midwives (**www.nmc.org.uk/standards/guidance/the-professional-duty-of-candour/read-the-professional-duty-of-candour/**).

A duty of candour has also been incorporated into the NHS Constitution and the Health and Social Care Act 2008.

The duty to report within the NHS Constitution

The Department of Health has introduced changes to the NHS Constitution for England that make it clear that all NHS workers have a duty to report poor practice or the mistreatment of those receiving care from the health service (DoH, 2015). It emphasises the following points:

(continued)

continued . . .

- *ensure that you are treated with courtesy and you receive appropriate support throughout the handling of a complaint; and that the fact that you have complained will not adversely affect your future treatment*
- *ensure that when mistakes happen or if you are harmed while receiving health care you receive an appropriate explanation and apology, delivered with sensitivity and recognition of the trauma you have experienced, and know that lessons will be learned to help avoid a similar incident occurring again*
- *ensure that the organisation learns lessons from complaints and claims and uses these to improve NHS services.*

(www.gov.uk/government/publications/the-nhs-constitution-for-england)

The duty to report within the Health and Social Care Act 2008 (Regulated Activities) Regulations 2014

This Act sets out fundamental standards in law of a clear baseline below which care must not fall, against which the Care Quality Commission (CQC) can take enforcement action against providers that do not meet this standard. Nurses in England have a further duty to report poor practice under the provisions of the Health and Social Care Act 2008. The CQC (2009) also imposes essential standards for quality and safety to ensure that the requirements of the Health and Social Care Act 2008 are met. Suitable arrangements must be in place to ensure that service users are safeguarded against the risk of abuse by:

- *taking reasonable steps to identify the possibility of abuse and prevent it before it occurs;*
- *responding appropriately to any allegation of abuse.*

Nurses are expected to contribute to the achievement of these essential standards, and the CQC has powers to take action where a service fails to meet these requirements. These standards include a memorandum of understanding with the NMC that allows for an exchange of information between the two bodies. If a CQC inspection finds evidence of poor practice by a nurse, it will pass the information on to the NMC for investigation.

Given the existing legal obligations on nurses to report poor practice, it is arguable as to whether a further *duty of candour* will improve the rate of reporting. Improvement in reporting rates will only happen when nurses are confident that they will not face recrimination or be victimised by colleagues and managers, and that their concerns about practice will be acted upon. Reporting poor practice remains a dilemma for nurses who are aware of their duties but are fearful of the recrimination and the potential effect on their career.

A survey by the Royal College of Nursing of 3,000 members (Laurance, 2011) found that nurses were more reluctant to report concerns than they were two years previously. Some 80 per cent of respondents had raised concerns relating to patient safety, but in almost half of cases no action was taken. One-third said they had been discouraged from complaining and only one-third felt confident that their employers would protect them if they did raise concerns (Laurance, 2011).

Activity 8.2	*Critical thinking*

In Chapter 4 we introduced Rawls' *veil of ignorance* – return to the chapter and reread the concept summary if you need to. Using this thought experiment one can consider the ethicality of very many different types of action with a special awareness of the impact of the decision on others (primarily because the 'other' could be you). Using the concept of the veil of ignorance, revisit a past experience in the care setting where you have been unhappy about the care given to a patient, only this time consider how the patient might feel if she or he knew what you knew – what it might have been like to have been 'an informed' patient. Now consider if your response to the situation met the standards of candour we have discussed here.

Since the answers to this activity are personal to you, there is no specimen answer at the end of the chapter.

Protection for staff reporting poor practice is provided by the Public Interest Disclosure Act 1998. Its provisions protect against dismissal or detriment in individuals making a protected disclosure in respect of specific types of wrongdoing or malpractice (Employment Rights Act 1996, section 47B). An employer cannot prevent a worker from making a protected disclosure through a gagging clause as part of the employment contract or other agreement.

However, protection only extends to detriment and victimisation by the employer. Detriment arising from bullying and recrimination from colleagues is not covered by the Public Interest Disclosure Act 1998. In *Fecitt and others* v *NHS Manchester (Public Concern at Work Intervening)* [2011], three nurses reported a colleague at the walk-in centre where they worked. Although their concern was found to be justified, no further action was taken against the member of staff. Relations among the staff at the centre deteriorated as a result, and their employing trust responded by taking action against those who had reported poor practice. All three claimed they had been victimised and treated in a detrimental way as a result of their disclosure. The Court of Appeal held that the employing Trust could not be held liable for the behaviour of individual members of staff towards those who report poor practice. The court found that, in contrast to equality law, which held individuals personally liable for their acts of victimisation against those pursuing a discrimination claim, there is no provision making it unlawful for individual members of staff to victimise those who report poor practice. As employers can only be liable for the unlawful acts of their workers, the claim could not succeed.

The impact of the Court of Appeal decision in *Fecitt and others* is to remove protection for those who report poor practice from victimisation by individual members of staff. It discourages nurses from reporting poor practice. It will greatly limit the impact of any duty of candour imposed on nursing staff. Unless the Public Interest Disclosure Act 1998 extends its protection to include detriment and victimisation by colleagues in the same way as the Equality Act 2010 does for discrimination cases, nurses will continue to be wary of reporting poor practice, despite their legal duty to do so.

Ethical leadership

The duty of candour requires staff to speak out about mistakes in treatment or care. An enhanced conception of the duty of candour could, however, mean that nurses or managers who obstruct staff from speaking out about poor care could face criminal charges, according to the recommendations in the Francis Report (2013). However, while it is important to apply the highest possible standards, if new duties are introduced it will be crucial to have strong leadership to ensure there is no unnecessary blame on individuals when they raise concerns.

What is clear is that organisations need to develop a level of ethicality which reaches up from the shop floor to the board room and beyond; how this might be achieved is difficult to know. Clearly in an organisation of the size and nature of the NHS, developing and sustaining a single culture are perhaps impossible to achieve, but the impact which individuals can have on the culture and behaviours within their own area of practice can be huge. One of the challenges of this book is for you, the student nurse, to develop an understanding of what ethics are and then to consider how you will develop and live by this understanding throughout the rest of your career – for many this will include a time when you are in a position to exercise influence on the way others behave in your team or organisation; you will be the leaders.

It is worth noting that the Francis Report was not the first of its type. In 2001, a public inquiry report into children's heart surgery at Bristol Royal Infirmary highlighted poor organisation, failure of communication, lack of leadership, paternalism and a failure to put patients at the centre of care (Kennedy, 2001; The Stationery Office, 2002). As in the Francis Report, prioritisation of financial and managerial targets rather than patient safety and wellbeing was evident.

Taking both the Bristol and Mid Staffordshire reports together, similarities indicate a weak or coercive leadership and insufficient or poorly trained staff creating a culture where flaws were hidden or ignored, bullying was prevalent and patients suffered. Those retaining a professional ethic describe suffering **moral distress** (McCarthy, 2013), where the gap between their moral vision and their actions – what they were actually able to do in the circumstances – widened. Some staff left and others became immune to what was going on around them.

Central to the issues raised in both reports is the lack of coherent professional and institutional values coupled with pervasive organisational systems that value certain kinds of ends, such as meeting quantitative targets (like waiting times). These issues contribute to focusing managers and leaders away from the important elements of the provision of direct patient care. Managers and leaders exert pressure on those they manage and lead and a culture which values targets over people emerges.

In Mid Staffs, upwards of 120 jobs, mostly nursing posts, were removed in order to make savings to secure Foundation status for the hospital. These redundancies led to untrained and inexperienced nurses taking charge of seriously ill patients for whom they had neither the clinical skills nor the emotional resilience to care. Against this background, the culture of care delivery slipped further and a culture which valued the achievement of targets continued to grow apace.

Activity 8.3 — *Reflection*

Consider the values which you identified back in Activity 1.5 (Chapter 1). These were the values which drew you to nursing in the first place, many of which you share with other students and trained nurses. Consider how you demonstrate these values in what you do and how you behave in the practice area. Now think about the manager in your most recent practice placement. How does this manager behave and how does s/he demonstrate the things s/he most values? Remembering that this manager has a broader agenda and remit than you as a student, reflect on how the two lists compare.

This activity is meant to help highlight some of the tensions which exist for nurses who also have to manage. Clearly both patient care and the management of staff and resources are important; it is how these translate into how the manager behaves which will set the tone for the culture of the team.

Both the Mid Staffs and Bristol reports portray organisations which value ends that can be tangibly measured (like waiting times) as well as organisations whose main concern is the measuring of those outcomes. This focus on measurable ends to quantify performance, rather than care, devalues healthcare to the level at which it becomes a mere matter of performing – where the practitioner works to meet imposed outcomes, rather than toward the central practice of healthcare, to provide care.

De Zulueta (2013) writes that many nurses are constrained in their work by the need to make efficiency savings. Prioritising efficiency savings over patient care makes nurses accountable to their general managers rather than to their professional bodies. This leads to a dissonance between the ideals of the profession, to care, and the measurable chosen ends of the organisation, to be efficient, and leads to a sense of moral distress in the nurses affected.

One of the key features of nursing ethics which distinguishes it from ethics per se, and medical ethics in particular, is the emphasis nursing ethics places on care, rather than cure. This emphasis on care reflects strongly on the belief of most nurses, that the relationship with the individual patient or client is as important as, if not more important than, what is actually done for and with the patient. This may seem like an odd thing to say at first until we consider the nature and scope of nursing practice. If we take any of the models of nursing, they point us to actions which are intended to support patients in their activities of daily living (Roper et al., 1980) to achieve independent living (Orem, 1991) or to learn to adapt (Roy and Andrews, 1999). These do not point to cure; they indicate a preoccupation with the human aspects of care, the sorts of things which are important for human flourishing – as we discussed in Chapter 1.

Ethical leadership in nursing has to take account of the need to support nurses in the attainment of these patient-centred nursing goals. The challenge posed here again is for nurses to remember, as they develop into a position where they can exert leadership, what the purpose of that leadership is. We would argue that the sole purpose of the ethically active nurse leader is to support the attainment of the shared purpose of nurses, the provision of care, through the ethical exercise of power and influence.

Professional and organisational values therefore need to be designed to enable clinical excellence, moral sensitivity, compassion and care and integrity. Empathy is intrinsic, as is the professional aspiration to do good for patients. For this, authentic leadership, strong teams, adequate staffing, a nurturing learning environment and willingness to acknowledge errors and to learn from them are essential.

Empirical ethics

It is reasonable to assume that most health professionals will have had some kind of ethics education in their training and to assume therefore that staff at Mid Staffs who would have had insight into the harm being caused would have known it to be unethical. If nurses had such insight, why did they not use it to prevent harm and do good? In part the answer to this lies in the fact that ethical theories do not always translate readily into everyday routine practice.

One of the problems with ethical theories, such as consequentialism and non-consequentialism (as examined in Chapter 4), for example, is that their applicability and usefulness in day-to-day activity are not always obvious. Second, consideration of ethics and the guidance which might derive from ethical considerations is low on the agendas of people who are occupied with the day-to-day business of care provision. So theories on their own do not necessarily make ethics useful to the individual nurse. Let's consider these points in some more detail:

- First, ethics provides a *theoretical* framework but does not necessarily explain how things *should* be done at the bedside. This distinction is therefore between knowing what *ought* to be done and understanding how care *is* being done. The difficulty for the application of ethics is in trying to traverse the distance between *ought* and *is*.
- Second, knowledge about ethics does not necessarily make individuals ethical practitioners. A person may act ethically, but may not be inherently ethical. Ethics therefore needs to be intrinsically inherent within the professional attributes and characteristics. So the old question remains – how do you make people want to be, and actually be, ethical?

In order for ethics to be useful in preventing harm and promoting good, we need to ask questions about how care is being done and how it ought to be done and we need to consider how individual nurses might become intrinsically ethical in their approach to their work.

One of the criticisms of ethics over the years is that it is just about theory and has little or no applicability to real life. In the final part of this chapter we will explore the concept of empirical ethics, which seeks to draw together an understanding of ethics and the real world; that is, it provides a model for us to carry some of the learning which has taken place in this book forward into our nursing practice.

Empirical inquiry into the concepts of ethics seeks to use research to uncover relationships between what is experienced in an ethical dilemma. Empirical ethics therefore explores what is actually experienced by people involved in the dilemma, which may show different understandings and perspectives about ethics, and these understandings may differ from the more abstract normative theories about ethics. This is important because the theories of ethics, such as consequentialism and deontology, attempt to describe the world as it *ought* to be, whereas empirical ethics uses research to explore and describe the world as it *is*, and considers it in relation to the *ought* (De Vries, 2001). For example, when looking at the workings of a health organisation, empirical research could explore how ethical leadership plays out at different levels in the organisation, such as at ward level or management level. This will describe how ethical leadership is being experienced by the workers in the organisation.

Empirical ethics therefore uses research to inquire into ethics as experienced. There are various approaches to 'doing' empirical ethics. Jacoby and Siminoff (2008) provide a useful means of grouping empirical work into four types.

Concept summary: empirical ethics

The first and most common type of empirical research is the linear model (Lindemann Nelson, 2000). These studies seek to define current practices, opinions and beliefs and can be descriptive or explanatory in nature. Such research might look at attitudes from different perspectives (e.g. nurses, physicians, patients and families), the efficacy of end-of-life care programmes or how people make difficult ethical choices. For example, such studies might ask questions such as: 'How many people are willing to make advance directives?' or 'How do people with chronic illness experience their illness?' (Lindemann Nelson, 2000).

The second approach is the social science critique. This type of research aims to demonstrate that the reality of practice does not always match the theoretical ideal. Here research explores the gaps between ethical ideals and the reality of healthcare. For example, research into medical errors found that care providers often fail to disclose errors to patients (Gallagher et al., 2006).

The third approach of empirical inquiry considers how to bring practice closer in line with ethical ideals. This type of research aims to design and test methods to help professionals care for patients in ways that are more consistent with ethical norms. For example, Dixon-Woods et al. (2007) demonstrated significant shortcomings in the use of many written-consent documents, raising the question of whether merely altering a form could ever sufficiently improve the consent process.

The final approach integrates research-based information into healthcare ethics (Haimes, 2002; Hedgecoe, 2004). This builds on the work of the previous three types of research through systematic analysis of multiple empirical publications to form the basis of an argument to change an ethical norm.

These approaches to empirical inquiry each have a purpose in the understanding of healthcare ethics, and importantly, they address the difference between the theories about ethics and the ethics as lived by the individual. When reading about ethics, it is important to think about how the literature has been informed. It is likely that you will read research-based papers about ethics in health practice, and these will likely be using one of the empirical ethics approaches detailed above. It is also important that you, as a developing nurse, develop the ability to use research-based literature to inform your understanding about ethics in relation to your practice.

Activity 8.4   *Evidence-based practice and research*

This is an activity for after, for now and the future, and one we hope you will find habit forming as you move forward into your nursing practice. Next time you come across an ethical issue in practice – such as resource allocation, truth telling or gaining informed consent – rather than just looking at the various opinion papers about what is the right or wrong thing to do, attempt to find some research in the area. Using your knowledge of research methodologies and methods, critically appraise the literature before you start to consider how it might be used to inform how you will act in the situation and similar situations in the future.

Since the answers to this activity are personal to you, there is no specimen answer at the end of the chapter.

The usefulness and power of research into ethical issues are the increasing mainstream nature of evidence-based nursing practice. Many commentators now include ethical consideration within their models of evidence-based nursing practice, demonstrating the importance of ethics as part of the decision-making process in practice (Ellis, 2016).

The importance of the use of empirical evidence in ethical decision making is undeniable. If we consider the arguments we have put forward in this book, most especially around letting the arguments guide our ethical and moral thinking (the inductive and reflective approach), then the need for nurses, and student nurses, to spend more time gathering evidence before responding to ethical issues becomes more apparent.

Evidence-based nursing

An essential aspect of the nursing role in delivering quality healthcare is based on information from available evidence. There are many reasons why nurses should engage in evidence-based practice. These include:

- the increasingly complex nature of healthcare decisions;
- the Department of Health's directive that services and treatments should be based on the best evidence of what does and does not work (DoH, 1997);
- compliance with codes of professional conduct;

- the nurse's ability to make informed judgements is of importance to patients and assists nurses in being valued members of multidisciplinary teams;
- nurses do not have the time to read extensively. The pragmatic process of appraising and using the literature benefits patients at the same time as expanding the nurses' knowledge base.

Sackett et al. (1996) define evidence-based practice as *the conscientious, explicit, and judicious use of current best evidence in making decisions about the care of individual patients.*

This definition emphasises clinical reasoning and as being informed by the best available evidence. This is important to think about, and simply having access to the latest research does not in itself constitute evidence-based practice. Rather, it is the appropriate and judicious use of the best information for the individual patient. This means the nurse needs to be able to determine what makes evidence credible and therefore useful to apply to practice. This means you need to develop and refine your skills continually to be able to search for, and assess, the credibility of published research in relation to your practice, and you are likely to engage in research critiquing within your continuing professional development. The ability to critique published research-based evidence is essential as indiscriminate use of evidence could lead to potential harm to the public. As such, it is integral within the nurse's role to develop the skills to appraise evidence critically before using it in practice.

In their practice therefore, nurses therefore have a threefold responsibility:

1. to be aware of the latest evidence;
2. to ensure that evidence is applicable to the particular healthcare setting and practice being undertaken;
3. to work with colleagues to implement evidence appropriately.

The ethicality of this approach is further underpinned by considerations of core ethical theme principles such as 'doing good' and 'avoiding harm' as well as utilitarian principles of maximising happiness; such ideals are best achieved when the interventions we apply as nurses are informed by evidence rather than rite or ritual.

Future considerations for ethical nursing

The Francis Report (2013) contains 290 recommendations addressed to different parts of the NHS from which action has been taken to develop openness and transparency in health and social care practices and professional regulation. While this is affirmative action, nurses need to engage and be ethically engaged and active in their professional duties. Nursing ethics is centrally placed to develop understandings about ethics, but the onus of responsibility in developing an ethical nursing profession is owned by nurses both individually and collectively.

Professional and institutional values need to coalesce, and organisational systems need to be designed to enable clinical excellence, moral sensitivity, compassion and care, integrity and wisdom to flourish. Empathy is intrinsic, as is the professional aspiration to do good for patients. We need to ensure the relational and moral dimensions of care – the recognition that illness involves change and sometimes suffering. For this, we need resonant and authentic leadership at all levels, strong teams, adequate staffing, a nurturing learning environment and willingness to acknowledge errors and to learn from them. As nurses we need to support each other and provide positive role models to all those we work with.

We need to value and respect the emotional labour and complexity involved in the work of nursing. Hospitals provide care to living human systems; they are not factories designed around standardised procedures that can be mechanistically and quantitatively measured. Systems of blame for differing disciplines and professional practices, and systems where nurses are not enabled to individually and collectively account for their care, need to be challenged by nurses. The duty of candour provides such a mechanism to challenge systems and practices that may cause harm. Empirical inquiry into our practices to illuminate practices and experiences of care and caring are powerful tools for nurses and nursing to use to develop the art and science of nursing, and most importantly, to protect the public from potential harms.

Activity 8.5 *Reflection*

Now that you have almost reached the end of the book, take some time to reflect on what you feel you have learned through reading it. Make a list of three or four points you feel will help you to be a more ethically aware nurse. How do you think you might integrate these into your practice?

Since the answers to this activity will be personal to you, there is no specimen answer at the end of the chapter.

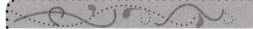

Chapter summary

This chapter has provided an overview of some of the issues which face nursing as an ethical undertaking now and which will continue to face nursing in the future. It has demonstrated the value of developing systems of care in which honesty and integrity are valued as much as the provision of care itself. We have explored some aspects of the role of the nurse as a leader of care and the duties attendant to that role.

In introducing empirical ethics we have added a further dimension to the challenge posed in this book, which has been about the need to approach ethical issues and dilemmas in the nursing in an inductive manner. The adoption of an approach to ethical decision making which is informed by experience, reflection, theory, practicality and research evidence will undoubtedly create some problems for many readers as this is both potentially confusing and time consuming.

(continued)

continued . . .

What is clear, however, is that the demographic, technological and political landscapes which drive healthcare policy and provision are rapidly changing and it is no longer acceptable for nurses either to ignore ethical issues claiming they are someone else's responsibility or to hide behind the provisions made within our codes of conduct. Instead the future for nursing and ethical nursing practice is one in which we will have to take responsibility for our actions and where the ethical justification of those actions will become increasingly complex.

Activities: brief outline answers

Activity 8.1 Decision making

In this scenario, Ruth has two issues about which she may need to be candid. The first issue is one for the care home itself and the need to address poor patient moving practices; this impacts on both staff and patient safety. The second is the bruising: while Ruth has no reason to believe the staff meant to bruise the patient, and indeed they were talking nicely to the patient and 'being helpful' as they saw it, the bruising does represent 'harm'. Ruth rightly decides she will discuss both issues with the care home manager, who thanks Ruth for bringing the issue to her attention. The care manager arranges extra training for the healthcare assistants and proactively seeks to explain the bruising to the patient's family, fulfilling her duty of candour.

Activity 8.3 Reflection

This is a challenging activity. You will have come up with one of three types of answer:

1. You can see there is a direct correlation between your values and the values which the manager displays. While you show care and attention to your patients, the manager does the same for the staff perhaps. Where you put the welfare of patients first and communicate openly and honestly with them, the manager is empathetic towards the staff and is interested in the welfare of patients.
2. You can see some similarities between the values you have and those of the manager. Perhaps the manager shows some interest in the patients' welfare and some in the welfare of staff but appears to be distracted by things which are not yet obvious to you. Perhaps the manager shuts him/herself off, either really or metaphorically, in order to undertake some tasks.
3. You cannot understand how the manager was ever a nurse or care professional. S/he is uninterested in the welfare of both staff and patients and puts the achievement of targets and the ticking of boxes above everything else.

Further reading

Ellis, P (2016) *Evidence Based Practice for Nurses*, 3rd edn. London: Sage.
More on the use of evidence in nursing deliberations.

Goleman, D, Boyatzis, RE and McKee, A (2002) *The New Leaders: Transforming the Art of Leadership into the Science of Reality*. London: Little, Brown.
Insights into ethical leadership from Goleman, the best-known writer on emotional intelligence.

Useful websites

www.businessballs.com/ethical_management_leadership.htm
Business balls is a quirky but sound website with leadership challenges; this page is on ethical leadership.

www.cebm.net/index.aspx?o=1023

The Centre for Evidence-Based Medicine is based at the University of Oxford. This website includes tools for identifying and critically appraising evidence.

www.cochrane.org

The Cochrane Collaboration is an international network that produces a library of Cochrane reviews, which are systematic reviews of primary research in healthcare and health policy.

www.evidence.nhs.uk

NHS Evidence provides accredited clinical and non-clinical local, regional, national and international information, including evidence, guidance and government policy.

www.mindtools.com/pages/article/newLDR_58.htm

Mind tools is a well-used website looking at leadership tools; this page is about ethical leadership.

www.rcn.org.uk/library

Royal College of Nursing library services and archives – one of the largest specialist nursing libraries in the world.

Glossary

Abortion   unless otherwise stated, as used in this book this refers to the termination of a pregnancy undertaken in the hospital setting.

Acculturation   adaptation of self to take on the beliefs and ways of acting which are prevalent in a new culture.

Act of commission   an action an individual chooses to do.

Act of omission   choosing not to do something.

Act utilitarianism   the actions which people do are only right if they maximise happiness in any given situation.

Active euthanasia   when some positive action is taken to bring about the death of the individual.

Actuality   when some potential has been achieved.

Advocacy   representing the views of another person as if they were one's own.

Advocate   someone who practises advocacy.

Aesthetic   judgements based on our sensory responses to something.

Agency   the ability of an individual to make choices.

Agent   a person who is exercising agency.

Anencephalic   congenital absence of some or all of the brain and spinal cord.

Autonomy   the ability to make choices about things which affect oneself; also called self-governance.

Beneficence   the principle of doing good.

Best interests   the notion that we are doing something for some greater good of an individual, some best interest of theirs.

Binary thinking in the sense used here, it refers to a way of defining your identity with reference to the differences between you and someone else; see **othering**.

Candour the duty to be open and honest when dealing with other people.

Capacity the mental ability of an individual to make choices.

Case law refers to the development of laws by the courts in response to real cases brought before them which then provide the basis for judgements in similar cases in the future.

Claim in rights terminology, a claim over how other people should act – in a negative claim by not interfering or in a positive claim by providing help.

Common law a system whereby law is generated and enacted in relation to prior judgements made in the legal setting.

Confidentiality protecting information which belongs to/is about another person and which that person has not given permission to share.

Congruence as used in this book, it means consistent or true to oneself.

Consent the process by which a person agrees to something.

Consequentialism a school of ethical thought concerned with the rightness of the outcome of an action.

Critical interests interests people have which relate to things which make human life worthwhile, like friendship and personal reputation.

Cultural norms Ways of being and behaving which are accepted as normal in a given culture

Decisional capacity the ability to make a decision but not necessarily to be able to act on it.

Deductive finding the evidence to support a predetermined hypothesis or understanding of how things should be.

Deontology/duty-based ethics the school of ethical thought which places emphasis on the rightness of the action being undertaken; also called **non-consequentialism**.

Determinism a view of the world which suggests our actions are predetermined – that is, they arise out of what went before; there is no free will.

Dialectic questioning wider political and social issues which frame the problem you are considering.

Dilemma   where there appear to be two or more equally correct ways of acting.

Doctrine of double effect   a Roman Catholic doctrine which helps justify the negative outcomes of an action by reference to the positive intentions which underlie the act itself.

Duty of care   that duty which applies to all healthcare professionals in relation to the patients they care for which arises out of the nature of the professional–patient relationship and is strongly associated with the existence of special rights.

Emotivism   a branch of ethical thinking sometimes associated with a positivist approach to knowledge which suggests all ethical decisions are merely matters of opinion because they cannot be tested by the senses. Emotivism justifies its ethical position by regarding human experience as a good grounding for ethical decision making.

Empirical ethics   ethical thought which is derived from research.

Empowerment   to give, or return, power to another person.

Ends in themselves   the practice of showing respect for persons rather than seeing people as a tool to achieving one's own aims.

Ethic of reciprocity   to 'do unto others as you would have them do to you', a rule recognised in many religions as well as the ethical work of Kant (see **golden rule** and **universality**).

Ethical congruence   see **congruence**.

Euthanasia   the act of taking a life, usually of a terminally ill person, in order to relieve that person's suffering. Literally means good death.

Experiential interests   interests which beings capable of suffering have and which relate to the avoidance of suffering.

Four principles approach   an approach to ethical decision making ascribed to Beauchamp and Childress which uses the notions of *doing good, avoiding harm, autonomy* and *justice* as the basis for ethical decision making in biomedicine.

Free will   the idea that humans are capable of exercising choice.

Functionalist   a view of the world (or society) which considers it to be constituted from different parts, all of which have a role to play in its functioning.

Golden rule   to 'do unto others as you would have them do to you', a rule recognised in many religions as well as the ethical work of Kant (see **ethic of reciprocity** and **universality**).

Human flourishing   after Aristotle, meaning to achieve the purpose in one's life/achieving ones full potential.

Human rights   rights which people have because they are human.

Human worth   the notion that being human is what confers people with their ethical and moral value.

Immunity   where no one can change the form of right the individual has.

Inductive   in the sense used in this book, allowing the ethical principles to guide our decision making rather than making up our mind and then finding the principles to underpin our opinion.

Intent/intention   the word used in ethics to describe the motivation for how we act. Before any action there is a thought process which decides on that action – it is the intent to act which drives the action itself.

Interests   in the ethical sense, these are the things which are important to and about people in general. A basic example might be an interest in avoiding pain; a more complex example might be an interest in maintaining personal dignity.

Involuntary euthanasia   when individuals cannot participate in the decision to euthanise them (e.g. because of dementia or coma).

Involuntary passive euthanasia   euthanasia in which the person has not been involved in the decision making because he or she is unable (e.g. in a coma) and in which the death is achieved through an act of omission.

Justice   fairness; treating people in similar circumstances in essentially the same way.

Liberty   in relation to rights, this means an individual has the right not to be interfered with but no claim to help from others.

Means to an end   treating other people as a tool to achieving one's own goals, rather than as ends in themselves.

Moral calculus   an idea from **utilitarianism** which suggests the goodness of an action can be calculated using an equation consisting of minimising pain and maximising pleasure.

Moral dilemma   where there is a moral tension between two or more courses of action.

Moral distress   distress which arises as a result of moral stress.

Moral stress   stress which arises when individuals find themselves acting in ways which are at odds (incongruent) with their personal beliefs and values.

Morally relevant   things which are of ethical and moral significance, such as the way people behave; this is as opposed to things which are not morally relevant, such as gender, age and ethnicity.

Narcissistic   concern with how the self appears to others; self-oriented.

Necessary condition   a condition which must be true if a corresponding something is also true.

Non-consequentialism   a school of ethical thought concerned with doing the right thing regardless of the consequences – see **deontology/duty-based ethics**.

Non-maleficence   avoiding doing harm. Or, more correctly, avoiding doing deliberate harm (or doing harm with a view to achieving a good outcome in the longer term).

Non-voluntary euthanasia   euthanasia against the person's will.

Normative ethics   the study of ethical action.

Ontological/ontology   the theory of being.

Othering   the process of defining who you are by reference to certain characteristics you possess which the 'other' does not; see **binary thinking**.

Parentalistic   a behaviour which a parent might engage in; treating someone like a child.

Passive euthanasia   allowing an individual to die even though that person's life might have been prolonged.

Persistent vegetative state   a coma-like state in which the person is 'alive' but has no level of conscious activity.

Person-centredness   viewing people as a unique person and focusing on this in your interaction.

Personhood   the characteristics which help define us as human.

Positivist/positivism   a school of thought which suggests we can only know things which we can see and test using our senses.

Positional power   power that someone has because of the position they hold or the job that they do.

Potentiality   the potential of a living person or foetus; potentiality may provide a basis for moral worth, e.g. we often grieve more over deaths in young people because of the loss of potential.

Power   in relation to rights, an individual has the ability to change the form of the right.

Practice-grounded   ways of understanding and working which are based on reflections on practice situations

Precedent   in the legal sense this relates to the fact that judgements have to be made which reflect those previously made where a case in law is substantially the same as one which has a previous judgement.

Prima facie   a term used in law and ethics which literally means at first sight. This refers to ideas, arguments or statements which appear correct on first (perhaps superficial) view.

Pro-choice   in this view personal **autonomy** and **self-determination** are more important than any other ethical consideration.

Pro-life   the argument that in ethical terms life should take precedence over everything else (e.g. abortion should not be allowed even if the women has the right to self-determination).

Respect for persons   the notion that we should act ethically towards other people because they are human.

Right to die   a right claimed by some people in the euthanasia debate suggesting that individuals have the right to be actively, or passively, euthanised if that is their wish.

Right to life   has various meanings depending on the context in which it is discussed, e.g. the foetal right not to be aborted; the right not to be murdered.

Rights   legal, or ethical, tools for protecting the individual from unwarranted, and unwanted, interference.

Rule utilitarianism   people should follow the rule which will lead to the greatest happiness.

Self-determination   having the moral status which allows individuals to make choices about their own life (see **agency** and **autonomy**).

Sick role   the functionalist theory which suggests patients are obliged to cooperate with professional care givers in order to get better again.

Special responsibilities   additional responsibilities we take on because we enter into special relationships, such as becoming a nurse, a spouse or a parent. That is, the responsibility exists because we chose to create and accept it.

Special rights   these exist in special relationships where an individual has agreed to accept special responsibility for something, such as the behaviours a patient can expect from a nurse but not from a checkout operator or bus driver.

Statute   law generated by a legislative body such as Parliament.

Sufficient condition   something which, if present, provides sufficient grounds to believe something else is true.

Transpersonal   considering how you are developing as a person.

Trump   as used in the book, trumps are reasons to overrule any other considerations.

Universality   to 'do unto others as you would have them do to you', a rule from the work of Kant also recognised in many religions (see **ethic of reciprocity** and **golden rule**).

Utilitarianism   a form of consequentialist thought where the outcomes of an action are seen to justify the action so long as the outcome is positive.

Values   beliefs which guide the way we behave (or would like to behave).

Virtue ethics/theory   a school of ethical thought concerned with the ethical character of individuals and the decisions they make.

Voluntary euthanasia   when an individual requests to be euthanised.

References

Adams, R (2006) *A Theory of Virtue: Excellence in Being for the Good*. Oxford: Oxford University Press.

Alkire, S (2007) Religion and development, in Clark, DA (ed.) *The Elgar Companion to Development Economics*. Cheltenham: Edward Elgar Publishing.

Allmark, P (1993) Euthanasia, dying well and the slippery slope. *Journal of Advanced Nursing*, 18: 1178–1182.

Allmark, P and Klarzynski, R (1992) The case against nurse advocacy. *British Journal of Nursing*, 2(1): 33–36.

Aristotle, translated by Thompson, JA (1976) *The Nicomachean Ethics*. London: Penguin.

Armstrong, AE (2006) Towards a strong virtue ethics for nursing practice. *Nursing Philosophy*, 7(3): 110–124.

Avery, G (2013) *Law and Ethics in Nursing and Healthcare: An Introduction*. London: Sage.

BBC (2016) Belgium minor first to be granted euthanasia. Available online at: /www.bbc.co.uk/news/world-europe-37395286 (accessed 30/12/2016)

Beauchamp, T and Childress, J (2012) *Principles of Biomedical Ethics*, 7th edn. Oxford: Oxford University Press.

Benjamin, M and Curtis, J (2010) *Ethics in Nursing*, 4th edn. Oxford: Oxford University Press.

Bentham, J (1781) *The Principles of Morals and Legislation*, published 1987. New York: Prometheus Books.

Blais, KK, Hayes, JS, (2015) *Professional Nursing Practice: Concepts and Perspectives*, 7th edn. Upper Saddle River, NJ: Pearson Education.

Bosshard, G and Materstvedt, LJ (2011) Medical and societal issues in euthanasia and assisted suicide, in Chadwick, R, ten Have, H and Meslin, EM (eds) *The Sage Handbook of Health Care Ethics*. London: Sage.

Brown, J, Stevens, J and Kermode, S (2012) Supporting student nurse professionalisation: the role of the clinical teacher. *Nurse Education Today*, 32(5): 606–610.

Care Quality Commission (2009) *Essential Standards of Quality and Safety*. Newcastle: CQC.

Christensen, M and Hewitt-Taylor, J (2006) Empowerment in nursing: paternalism or maternalism? *British Journal of Nursing*, 15(13): 695–699.

Cox, K, Bird, L, Arthur, A, Kennedy, S, Pollock, K, Kumar, A, Stanton, W and Seymour, J (2013) Public attitudes to death and dying in the UK: a review of published literature. *British Medical Journal: Supportive & Palliative Care*, 3: 37–45.

Davies, C (2003) *Workers, Professions and Identity*, in Henderson, J and Atkinson, D (eds.) *Managing Care in Context*. Milton Keynes: Open University Press.

Department of Health (1997) *The New NHS: Modern, Dependable*. London: Department of Health.

De Vries, R (2001) The fact of bioethics: a comment on Peter Singer. *Society*, 38(5): 36–40.

De Zulueta, P (2013) Reflecting on the Francis Report: how can we develop more human systems of care? *Nursing Ethics*, 20: 838–840.

Dixon-Woods, M, Booth, A and Sutton, AJ (2007) Synthesising qualitative research: a review of published reports. *Qualitative Research*, 73: 375–422.

Dresser, R (2010) Dworkin on dementia: elegant theory, questionable policy, in Kuhse, H and Singer, P (eds) *Bioethics: An Anthology*, 2nd edn. Oxford: Blackwell.

Dworkin, G (1988) *The Theory and Practice of Autonomy*. New York: Cambridge University Press.

Dworkin, R (1987) *Taking Rights Seriously*, 5th edn. London: Duckworth.

Dworkin, R (1992) Rights as trumps, in Waldron, J (ed.) *Theories of Rights*. Oxford: Oxford University Press.

Dworkin, R (1993) *Life's Dominion: An Argument about Euthanasia and Abortion*. London: Harper Collins.

Dyer, V (2002) Diane Pretty makes final 'death with dignity' plea. *The Guardian*. Available online at: http://www.theguardian.com/society/2002/mar/20/health.uknews (accessed 17/06/2014).

Eby, MA (2000) Producing evidence ethically, in Gomm, R and Davies, C (eds) *Using Evidence in Health and Social Care*. London: Sage.

Ellis, P (1992) Tony Bland: living a dilemma. *Nursing Standard*, 7(12): 41–43.

Ellis, P (1996) Exploring the concept of acting 'in the patient's best interests'. *British Journal of Nursing*, 5(17): 1072–1074.

Ellis, P (2012) Rights and responsibilities, in Koubel, G and Bungay, H (eds) *Rights, Risks and Responsibilities – Interprofessional Perspectives*. Basingstoke: Palgrave.

Ellis, P (2016) *Evidence-Based Practice in Nursing*, 3rd edn. London: Sage.

Emanuel, EJ and Miller, FG (2007) Money and distorted ethical judgment about research: ethical assessment of the TeGenero TGN1412 trial. *American Journal of Bioethics*, 7: 76–81.

English, J (1984) Abortion and the concept of a person, in Feinberg, J (ed.) *The Problem of Abortion*. Belmont, TN: Wadsworth.

Estefan, A (2011) Moral and ethical practice, in McAllister, M and Lowe, JB (eds) *The Resilient Nurse: Empowering Your Practice*. New York: Springer Publications.

Fecitt and others v *NHS Manchester* (Public Concern at Work Intervening) [2011] lj EWCA Civ 1190.

Finlay, L (2008) *Reflecting on 'Reflective Practice'*. Available online at: www.open.ac.uk/opencetl/sites/www.open.ac.uk.opencetl/files/files/ecms/web-content/Finlay-(2008)-Reflecting-on-reflective-practice-PBPL-paper-52.pdf (accessed 18/10/2016).

Francis, R (2013) *Report of the Mid Staffordshire NHS Foundation Trust Public Inquiry*. Available online at: www.midstaffspublicinquiry.com/report (accessed 04/05/2014).

Fry, S, Veatch, R and Taylor, C (2011) *Case Studies in Nursing Ethics*, 4th edn. London: Jones and Bartlett.

Gallagher, TH, Waterman, AD and Garbutt, JM (2006) US and Canadian physicians' attitudes and experiences regarding disclosing errors to patients. *Archives of Internal Medicine*, 16615: 1605–1611.

Gracia, D (2011) Deliberation and consensus, in Chadwick, R, ten Have, H and Meslin, EM (eds) *The Sage Handbook of Health Care Ethics*. London: Sage.

Haimes, E (2002) What can the social sciences contribute to the study of ethics? Theoretical, empirical and substantive considerations. *Bioethics*, 16(2): 89–113.

Hart, HLA (1992) Are there any natural rights? in Waldron, J (ed.) *Theories of Rights*. Oxford: Oxford University Press.

Hedgecoe, AM (2004) Critical bioethics: beyond the social science critique of applied ethics. *Bioethics*, 18(2): 120–143.

Henderson, V (1966) *The Nature of Nursing*. London: Macmillan.

HM Government (1929) *Infant Life (Preservation) Act 1929*. Available online at: www.legislation. gov.uk/ukpga/Geo5/19–20/34/section/1 (accessed 25/05/2014).

HM Government (1967) *The Abortion Act 1967*. Available online at: www.legislation.gov.uk/ ukpga/1967/87/contents (accessed 25/05/2014).

HM Government (1990) *Human Fertilisation and Embryology Act 1990*. Available at: www.legislation. gov.uk/ukpga/1990/37/contents (accessed 25/05/2014).

Hobbes, T (1651) edited by Tuck, R (1991) *Leviathan*. Cambridge: Cambridge University Press.

Hodkinson, K (2008) How should a nurse approach truth-telling? A virtue ethics perspective. *Nursing Philosophy*, 9(4): 248–256.

Hohfeld, WN (1919) *Fundamental Legal Conceptions as Applied in Judicial Reasoning*. New Haven, CT: Yale.

Howatson-Jones, L (2015) *Patient Assessment and Care Planning in Nursing*. London: Sage.

Howatson-Jones, L (2016) *Reflective Practice in Nursing*, 3rd edn. London: Sage.

Jacoby, L and Siminoff, L (2008) Empirical methods for bioethics: a primer, in Baker, R and Shelton, W (eds) *Advances in Bioethics*. Oxford: Elsevier Press.

Jeffreys, MR (2012) *Nursing Student Retention: Understanding the Process and Making a Difference*, 2nd edn. New York: Springer.

Jiga-Boy GM, Maio, GR, Haddock, G and Tapper, K (2016) Values and Behaviour, in Brosch, T and Sander, D (eds) *Handbook of Value: Perspectives From Economics, Neuroscience, Philosophy, Psychology and Sociology*. Oxford: Oxford University Press

Johns, C (2006) *Engaging Reflection in Practice: A Narrative Approach*. Oxford: Blackwell Publishing.

Johnstone, MJ (2009) *Bioethics: A Nursing Perspective*, 5th edn. London: Churchill Livingstone.

Kant, I (1785) translated by Gregor, M (1991) *The Metaphysics of Morals*. Cambridge: Cambridge University Press.

Kennedy, I (2001) *The Report of the Public Inquiry into the Children's Heart Surgery at the Bristol Royal Infirmary 1984–1995: Learning from Bristol.* Available online at http://webarchive. nationalarchives.gov.uk/+/www.dh.gov.uk/en/Publicationsandstatistics/Publications/ PublicationsPolicyAndGuidance/DH_4005620 (accessed 17/06/2014).

Laurance, J (2011) NHS whistleblowing safeguards not working. *Independent,* 5 December: 7.

Levenbook, BB (1984) Harming someone after his death. *Ethics,* 94: 407–419.

Lindemann Nelson, J (2000) Moral teachings from unexpected quarters: lessons for bioethics from the social sciences and managed care. *Hastings Centre Report,* 281: 12–17.

Luft, J and Ingham, H (1955) The Johari window, a graphic model of interpersonal awareness, in *Proceedings of the Western Training Laboratory in Group Development.* Los Angeles: UCLA.

Lützén, K, Cronqvist, A, Magnusson, A and Andersson, L (2003) Moral stress: synthesis of a concept. *Nursing Ethics,* 10: 312–322.

Lynch, J (2011) *Consent to Treatment.* Oxford: Radcliffe Publishing.

McCarthy, J (2013) Nursing ethics and moral distress: the story so far. *Nursing Ethics,* 20(2): 1–7.

Melia, K (2014) *Ethics for Nursing and Healthcare Practice.* London: Sage.

Mill, JS (1789) *Utilitarianism,* published 1990. Glasgow: Fontana Press.

Muir, N (2004) Clinical decision-making: theory and practice. *Nursing Standard,* 18(36): 47–52.

National Health Service, England (2015) The National Health Service (Revision of NHS Constitution Guiding Principles) Regulations 2015 available online at: www.legislation.gov.uk/ uksi/2015/1426/made (accessed 27/02/2017)

NHS Digital (2014) NHS Written Complaints Data released. Available online at: http://content. digital.nhs.uk/article/3414/NHS-written-complaints-data-released (accessed 17/10/2016)

Nursing and Midwifery Council (2007) *Fitness to Practise Annual Report: 1 April 2006 to 31 March 2007.* London: NMC.

Nursing and Midwifery Council (2015) *The Code: Professional Standards of Practice and Behaviour for Nurses and Midwives.* London: NMC.

Orem, DE (1991) *Nursing: Concepts of Practice,* 4th edn. St Louis, MO: Mosby-Year Book.

Parsons, T (1951) *The Social System.* London: Routledge and Kegan Paul.

Plato, translated by Lee, D (1981) *The Republic,* 2nd edn. London: Penguin Classics.

Rachels, J (1975) Active and passive euthanasia. *New England Journal of Medicine,* 292: 78–80.

Rachels, J (1993) Euthanasia, in Regan, T (ed.) *Matters of Life and Death: New Introductory Essays in Moral Philosophy,* 3rd edn. London: McGraw-Hill.

Rawls, J (1999) *A Theory of Justice,* revised edn. Oxford: Oxford University Press.

Rietjens, JAC, van Tol, DG, Schermer, M and van der Heide, A (2009) Judgement of suffering in the case of a euthanasia request in the Netherlands. *Journal of Medical Ethics,* 35(8): 502–507.

Roper, N, Logan, WW and Tierney, AJ (1980) *The Elements of Nursing.* Edinburgh: Churchill Livingstone.

Roy, C and Andrews, AA (1999) *The Roy Adaptation Model*, 2nd edn. Norwalk, CT: Appleton and Lange.

Sackett, D, Rosenberg, W, Gray, M, Haynes, R and Richardson, W (1996) Evidence based medicine: what it is and what it isn't. *British Medical Journal*, 312(7023): 71–72.

Sawyer, P (2014) Hero's welcome for runaway D-Day veteran. *The Telegraph*, 7 June. Available online at: www.telegraph.co.uk/history/world-war-two/10883278/Heros-welcome-for-runaway-D-Day-veteran.html (accessed 14/06/2014).

Schwartz, L (2002) Is there an advocate in the house? The role of health care professionals in patient advocacy. *Journal of Medical Ethics*, 28: 37–40.

Schwartz, SH (1992) Universals in the content and structure of values: theoretical advances and empirical tests in 20 countries, in Zanna MP (ed.) *Advances in Experimental Social Psychology*. London: Academic Press.

Schwartz, SH (1994) Are there universal aspects in the structure and contents of human values? *Journal of Social Issues*, 50: 19–45.

Select Committee on Science and Technology (2007) *Twelfth Report*. Available online at: www.publications.parliament.uk/pa/cm200607/cmselect/cmsctech/1045/104505.htm (accessed 18/05/2014).

Singer, P (1986) All animals are equal, in Singer, P (ed.) *Applied Ethics*. Oxford: Oxford University Press.

Singer, P (2011) *Practical Ethics*, 3rd edn. Cambridge: Cambridge University Press.

Slowther, A (2002) Special clinical ethics symposium: the case of Ms B and the 'right to die'. *Journal of Medical Ethics*, 28(4): 243.

Stanford Dictionary of Philosophy (2013) Available online at: http://plato.stanford.edu (accessed 03/05/2014).

Stationery Office (2002) *Learning from Bristol: The Department of Health's Response to the Report of the Public Inquiry into Children's Heart Surgery at the Bristol Royal Infirmary 1984–1995*. London: The Stationery Office. Available online at: http://webarchive.nationalarchives.gov.uk/20130107105354/http://www.dh.gov.uk/prod_consum_dh/groups/dh_digitalassets/@dh/@en/documents/digitalasset/dh_4059479.pdf (accessed 17/06/2014).

Stationery Office (2005) Mental capacity Act 2005. London: The Stationery Office. Available online at: www.legislation.gov.uk/ukpga/2005/9 (accessed 19/10/2016)

Sulmasy, DP and Pellegrino, ED (1999) The role of the double effect: cleaning up the double talk. *Archives of Internal Medicine*, 159: 545–550.

Taft, SH and White, J (2007) Ethics education: using inductive reasoning to develop individual, group, organizational and global perspectives. *Journal of Management Education*, 31(5): 614–646.

Thomson, JJ (1971) A defence of abortion. *Philosophy and Public Affairs*, 1(1): 47–66.

Timmins, F (2006) Critical practice in nursing care: analysis, action and reflexivity. *Nursing Standard*, 20(39): 49–54.

Titchen, A and McMahon, A (2013) Practice development as radical gardening: enabling creativity and innovation, in McCormack, B, Manley, K and Titchen, A (eds) *Practice Development in Nursing and Healthcare*, 2nd edn. Chichester: Wiley-Blackwell.

Tooley, M (1972) Abortion and infanticide. *Philosophy and Public Affairs*, 2(1): 37–65.

Vavasseur, C, Foran, A and Murphy, JFA (2007) Consensus statements on the borderlands of neonatal viability: from uncertainty to grey areas. *Irish Medical Journal*, 100(8): 561–564.

Wainwright, P (1991) Do nurses have ethics? *Nursing Standard*, 5(31): 46–47.

Warren, MA (1973) On the moral and legal status of abortion. *The Monist*, 57(4): 43–61.

Wellington, B and Austin, P (1996) Orientations to reflective practice. *Educational Research*, 38(3): 307–316.

Woodard Leners, D (1992) Intuition in nursing practice: deep connections. *Journal of Holistic Nursing*, 10(2): 137–153.

Index

National Health Service (NHS) *cont.*
  contract 9
  duty to report 133–4
natural rights 7
necessary conditions 112, **149**
non-consequentialism 59–60, **149**
  pros and cons 65
non-judgemental 58
non-maleficence 61–2, **149**
non-voluntary euthanasia 121, **149**
normative ethics 55, **149**
nursing
  importance of 8
  values 11–12
  see also The Code; ethical nursing
Nursing and Midwifery Council (NMC)
  and confidentiality 84
  and conscientious objection 118
  Standards for Pre-registration Nursing Education 6, 10,
    91, 131–2
  see also The Code

ontological questions 113, **149**
othering 15, 17, 100, **149**
outcome-focused nature of nursing 58

pain 48, 56, 94, 113, 119, 122, 125–6
parentalistic 94, **149**
Parsons, T. 92
participatory dialogue 30
passive euthanasia 119–20, **149**
Pellegrino, E.D. 125
persistent vegetative state 120, **149**
person-centredness 23, 89, **149**
personal ethics 6
personal values 11–13
personhood 88–9, 111–12, **149**
  necessary/sufficient conditions 112
  see also moral status of the foetus
phronesis 66
Plato 6
Poddar, Prosenjit 84–5
positional power 9, 23–4, 31, 100, **149**
positivist/positivism 48, **149**
potentiality 115, 116, **149**
Powelson, Dr 84
power 11, 48, 100, **149**
  empowerment 91–3, 94, **147**
  positional power 9, 23–4, 31, 100
practicality 49
practice-grounded understanding 22, **149**
precedents 42, **150**
prejudice 40
Pretty, Diane 123
prima facie justification 122, **150**
pro-choice 111, 122–3, **150**
pro-life 110, 111, 124–5, **150**
professional codes 9, 45
  see also The Code
professional ethics 6
professional identities 13–14, 15, 18

professional values 10, 11–13, 136, 141–2
Public Interest Disclosure Act (1998) 135

Rachels, J. 54, 124
Rawls, J. 63, 135
reciprocity, ethic of 60, **147**
reflection 1, 21–3
  case study 23–4
  critical reflection 27
  developing ethical values 24–8
  dialectic reflection 24
  ethical problem solving 30–3
  transpersonal reflection 24–5
reflexive responses 27, 28–30
reflexivity 22
relativism 49–50
religion 38, 41, 45–6, 59, 124
research
  critique 28–9
  empirical research 139–40, 141
respect for autonomy 44, 64, 65, 89–91, 98
respect for dignity 16, 65, 89
respect for humanity 16
respect for persons 14–16, 17–18, 32, 65, 90, 95,
    98, **150**
'right thing to do' 54
right to confidentiality 83–5
right to die 122–3, **150**
right to health 76
right to healthcare 76
right to life 7, **150**
right to refuse treatment 46, 74
right to self-preservation 7
rights 2, 71–3, **150**
  arguments in abortion 116–17
  basis of rights 74–5
  case study 74
  claim 73, 74, 82–4
  and equality 83
  as ethical tools 73
  function of rights 73–4
  human rights 7–8, 72, 76–8
  and interests 78–82
  legal rights 75
  natural rights 7
  operation of rights 82–3
  special rights 8, 72, 75–6
Roman Catholicisim 38, 46, 125–6
Royal College of Nursing 134
rule-based theories 59–60
rule utilitarianism 57, 116, **150**

Sackett, D. *et al.* 141
safety 132
Saldanha, Jacintha 84
Schwartz, S.H. 11
scope 42, 64
Scott, Dr Richard 41, 45
self-awareness 25–6, 28–9
self-declaration (and *The Code*) 132–3
self-determination 62, 111, **150**

sentimentality 46–8
Shipman, Dr Harold 50
sick role 92, **150**
Siminoff, L. 139
Singer, P. 49, 79
social contracts 7–8, 9
social identity 15
social norms 44
social science critique 139
Socrates 6, 17
special responsibilities 8–9, **150**
special rights 8, 72, 75–6, **150**
staff management 137
statute law 42, 75, **150**
subjectivism 49–50
suffering 119, 120, 121–2
sufficient conditions 112, **150**
Suicide Act (1961) 124
Sulmasy, D.P. 125
support 3

Taft, S.H. 24
Tarasoff, Tatiana 84–5
theories of ethics 2, 52–3, 138, 139
    approaches to ethics 53–5
    consequentialism 55–9, 119
    four principles approach 60–4
    non-consequentialism 59–60, 65
    rule-based theories 59–60
    scope 42, 64
    virtue theory 65–8
Thomson, J.J. 116
time 27

Tooley, M. 115
transpersonal reflection 24–5, **151**
treatment, right to refuse 46, 74
trumps 73, **151**

understanding 98–9
Universal Declaration of Human Rights (1948)
    77–8
universal requirements 11
universality 59, 78, **151**
utilitarianism 56, 116, **151**
    act utilitarianism 56, 116
    rule utilitarianism 57, 116

values 6, 10–11, **151**
    case study 23–4
    defined 11–12
    developing ethical values 24–8
    institutional values 136, 141–2
    personal values 11–13
    professional values 10, 11–13, 136, 141–2
veil of ignorance 63, 135
victimisation 135
virtue theory 65–8, **151**
    excellence 66, 67
    moral character 65
    philosophical basis of 65
voluntary euthanasia 120, **151**
vulnerability 62–3

Wainwright, P. 18
Warren, M.A. 115
White, J. 24

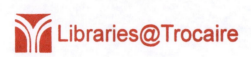